7 MINUTE
FITNESS STRENGTH
TRAINING
FOR SENIORS AND
OVER 60+

SIMPLE HOME EXCERCISE TO MAINTAIN
HEALTHIER BODY AND HIGH ENERGY IN
7 DAYS

LIAM OWEN

TABLE OF CONTENTS

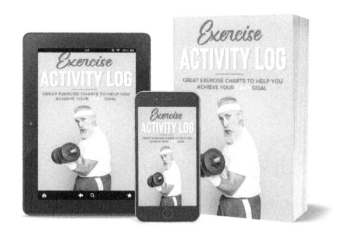

A SPECIAL GIFT TO OUR READERS!

Included with your purchase of this book is our **Exercise Activity Log** that will help you achieve your 7-day strength training goal. This is a great way to keep a record of your training.

USE THE LINK:
www.7minutestraining.com

OR SCAN THE QR CODE

JOIN OUR ONLINE SUPPORT GROUP

To maximize the value of your strength training, I highly encourage you to join our tight-knit community on Facebook, where you will be able to ask questions and get tips on your training.

USE THE LINK:

https://www.facebook.com/groups/strengthtrainingforseniors

OR SCAN THE QR CODE

The Day I Decided to Live.

I have always loved sports. I was an avid jogger in my youth, and I also enjoyed golf and soccer. As my years got the better of me, I adapted to a sedentary lifestyle. My kids went out in the world and made names for themselves. After my wife passed, I had a phase where I stopped taking care of myself. I didn't realize how bad things were until the day my son took me golfing. I just managed to arch my back into position before I fell flat on the golf course, writhing in pain. I was rushed to the emergency with a herniated disc.

That day changed a lot of things for me. I'd become used to getting by alone, but I noticed small omissions here and there. I forgot to turn the gas off after making my tea. I couldn't recall news events from the day before. And there was this constant, gnawing pain all over my body like I was stuck to one spot and could not move.

My sons began worrying about moving me to an assisted living facility. That was when I pulled my socks up. I wasn't having that! I still had some years left, and I meant to live each day of them as best as I could. So, I charted an exercise plan for myself.

You might laugh if I tell you that all it took was seven minutes every day. But, try it because these seven minutes changed my life. I can score Eagles at golf now. I play cricket with my kids and take my grandkids swimming on the weekends. I remember things my sons forget. And, I feel good.

Our bodies were not meant to be rooted to a spot, wasting away in front of screens. All it may take is seven minutes of your time - seven minutes to give you the life you deserve.

Understanding Older Adults

Older adults have to deal with a lot more than just alterations in their physical capabilities and cognitive strength. We may be adjusting to the passing of our friends and loved ones, struggling with finding a purpose to existence, adjusting to retirement, or be caught up caring for frail family members of the same age or older than ourselves. In 2005, a group of researchers remarked that negative emotions and feelings of depression were some of the top five reasons for reduced activity in older adults, whether they were exercisers or non-exercisers (Lees et al., 2005).

What Are We Afraid Of?

When it comes to physical activity, enjoying what we do is important. This becomes easier when we have social support and are fortified by believing that the exercise we do affects us positively. There can also be perceived barriers that get in the way of how much we exercise. For example, while some of us may think that exercise will positively affect our health, others believe that it isn't worth the effort, and we don't want to wake up and wheeze and huff for five to ten minutes for no good reason.

Some of us also become afraid that increased physical activity at old age may have adverse effects, like making us lose balance or increasing our palpitations. You see, these are perceived barriers. There's no telling if they will actually happen- but we use them to stop ourselves from getting up and moving. Take it as a kind of negative reinforcement. Remember when we were in school, and there were times that we didn't study for an exam because we were so confident we would do badly regardless of what we did? This is no different from that. The barriers are in our heads- and they can result from several reasons, one being the fear of not succeeding and remaining stuck in the same place regardless of how much effort we invest.

Here's what you need to know. There have been decades of epidemiological, clinical, and laboratory-based research regarding the role of physical activity in our lives. All have pointed to the importance of its regularity as a functional determinant of our physical health and well-being. In simple words, the more you move, the happier you will be (King, 2001).

A lot of things can go wrong when you stop physical activity. You can become a victim of the frailty syndrome, which refers to an overall decline of your health and functionality as you age; you can develop muscle strains and become prone to arthritis, chronic fatigue, and carpal tunnel. Now, while our desire to be a hundred percent certain of the positive effects of something before we launch into it often undoes us, there are other determinants when it comes to exercise.

You are Not Alone

A lot of problems among older adults stem from a lack of understanding of where to begin. How do we find the correct exercises? Which guides will work, and which will not? To top it off, we cannot schedule workouts because we don't know where to begin. Some of us, particularly those who don't have a background in fitness, are more susceptible to injuries, which gives rise to fear of falls and injuries.

Another issue with those who are new to the world of exercise is that people don't know how to start. This is natural- when we begin anything new, it's meant to feel overwhelming at the start. There are exercise plans out there that are too complicated or require expensive equipment, and they scare us off even before we can begin. It's also far easier to stick with a lack of motivation than to program ourselves to change. For people with athletic backgrounds like golfers, years of inactivity lead to problems with their abilities to play.

For those of us who have suffered injuries or accidents, the fears become greater and, at a level, affect us psychologically. Becoming weaker after multiple injuries and hospitalizations takes a lot from us and leaves us with a feeling of despair and incapacity. We feel internally fragile and consider relying on walking devices to get by.

Finding Your Mojo

An individual's motivational inclination to follow an exercise regimen may depend upon physical activity levels across several different demographics. For instance, a population-based study conducted on 286 Australian women between 50-64 years of age concerning their motivational readiness to exercise reported that those who did not benefit fit one stereotype. They had low knowledge of exercise, expected few psychological benefits from it, and had little to no family support compared to older women who were already exercising regularly (Lee, 1993).

As I mentioned before, there was also fear of injury, a perceived lack of ability, and the general belief that exercise had to be stressful or uncomfortable for it to be effective. Because of our preconceived notions, we are losing our identities, suffering poor health, and being burdened with alarming health care expenses.

I have been in your shoes. As older adults, we are up against a whole lot more when it comes to exercise. In general we lack confidence when it comes to our capabilities to complete tasks. As we age, we begin thinking that we are frail and give in to a sedentary lifestyle, which adds to further gaps in the way we perceive our bodies. We are afraid of falling, getting hurt, and making fools of ourselves. To top it off, we often become more apathetic to life as we age, and we look at things like exercise as boring. We cannot find the energy that we need to move, and instead, we huddle on a sofa with a book and a cup of tea.

But, here's the funny thing! Exercising could improve or reverse the conditions that keep you from taking up physical activity, to begin with! It can make you stronger, improve your locomotive abilities and balance, cure your depression, help you find a community, and improve your body image! Studies have shown that older adults across different ethnicities have reported improved productivity, increased self-esteem, elevated mood, and more robust overall health due to increased physical activity (Matthews et al., 2010)! Exercising can reduce the risks of falling and developing chronic complications like heart diseases, diabetes, cancer, and osteoporosis. It can improve the quality of life for those in poor health or disabled, increase self-validation, and reduce anxiety and depression (Matthews at al., 2010).

What Will You Take Away From This?

I am here to tell you that you have what it takes to lead a healthy, happy life. You have the power, the capabilities, and the faculties. I am a health writer and researcher with years of experience advising and training seniors on the correct exercise methods to combat aging. I have helped my family members lead fit, active lifestyles because learning begins at home. I have dedicated my life to fitness research for older adults and discussing and writing about human performance, injury prevention, and rehabilitation. I am here to help you take control of your life.

As we go deeper into the book, we will discuss the relationship between your age and physical health, the benefits of exercising, and common misconceptions that stop people of our age from taking up a form of activity. I will give you simple exercise routines that will take seven minutes of your time. We will also discuss a seven-day strength-training plan that will revitalize you and allow you to enjoy your life truly.

You will notice that the workout plans and exercises are simple and easy to follow if you keep up. They will take a few minutes of your day and leave you with knowledge and practice in order to strengthen your muscles and improve your mobility and stability. This will keep you from losing balance. The exercises can be done at home, and you don't need any extra equipment. They are straightforward, and I will take you through each step so that you have no trouble learning them.

You will also learn easy ways to boost your energy without relying on medication and unhealthy energy-boosting drinks loaded with artificial flavor and sugar. You will recover from injuries better, and you may develop so much mobility that you don't need walking devices any longer!

The ultimate purpose is to provide you with dependable and beneficial exercises to include in your daily life so that you can lead a healthier, stronger independent, and pain-free life! I will accompany you through this journey, hoping that it helps you realize that you don't need expensive equipment or fifty pounds of muscle to get up and get moving. All you need is functional limbs and faith. If you haven't downloaded my 7-day strength training log then you can do so by going to **www.7minutestraining.com**

So, let us begin with the full intent that by the time we are done, we will not just say but also believe that "age is just a number!" We cannot control the numbers, but we can control how we age. This can change so much for us, and to age well, we need to be active. Whether we are above forty or above sixty, we can always take control of our lives and improve our health and fitness levels. Do not give up hope or accept the decline of your health as a natural process. If you can include these small changes in your daily life, everything will start improving, and you will find that you are enjoying every second of your existence.

CHAPTER 1

Old Age and Physical Health

Let us understand how aging works for humans. At the biological level, aging results from an accumulation of molecular and cellular degradation over time. This doesn't just happen at the physical level. Our bodies are programmed to change, right down to our cells. As our cells age, their functions become slower. Eventually, old cells die as part of the body's normal function. Some old cells die because they are pre-programmed to do so. This programmed death is apoptosis, a kind of cell suicide that allows old cells to make room for new ones.

Old cells also die because they cannot multiply any longer. Our genes predetermine the multiplication limit. When cells can no longer divide, they grow larger, exist for a while, and perish. The cell division limit mechanism involves a structure called a telomere. Each time a cell divides, the telomeres shorten. Eventually, they become too short to make room for division. When a cell cannot divide any further, we have senescence. This is a natural outcome of age.

An evolutionary explanation behind the mystery of aging is based on individual fitness and selection, not group selection. This was propagated during the 1940s and 1950s by evolutionary biologists Haldane, Medawar, and Williams, who studied and reported that aging is simply an evolutionary outcome of a natural selection becoming inefficient at maintaining function and fitness during old age. In other words, the less physically fit we are, the frailer we become. From this perspective, aging becomes much more than a number. It involves the degradation that goes on in our bodies due to our lack of effort at maintaining our fitness (Fabian & Flatt, 2011).

Why You Matter

According to data released by the World Health Organization, people worldwide are living longer. A healthy, functional adult can expect to live into their sixties and beyond in this current age. By 2050, the world's aged population (60 years and older) is expected to increase to 2 billion. There are around 125 million people that are aged 80 years or older. By 2050, there will be 434 million people in this age group worldwide (Ageing and Health, 2018).

A longer life comes with a host of opportunities. These don't just extend to older people and their families, but to whole societies. Additional years allow us to pursue new activities such as further education, a new job, or pursuing a passion that we haven't had time for. This contributes to the well-being of a whole society and its intellectual development. I tell every older person never to underestimate the value you have to society. So, how can we ensure that you are a holistic component of it, along with being an individual in your own right? *By ensuring that you are in good health.*

Exercising and Its Effects on Human Muscles

If you have crossed 60, we need to be talking about muscle care. Nearly a quarter of all adults over the age of 60, and half of those over 80, have thinner arms and legs than what they did in their youth.

In 1988, Irwin Rosenberg, a faculty of Nutrition and Medicine at Tufts University, coined the term *sarcopenia.* The term was used to describe the deterioration of flesh (muscles) with age. Now, muscle aging probably has several fundamental causes. This includes decreasing numbers of muscle stem cells, mitochondrial dysfunction, a decline in the quality of protein absorption and turnover by the body, and hormonal deregulation (Butler-Browne et al., 2018).

Loss of muscle mass can be preceded by muscle fatigue and weakness, making us feel tired to perform menial daily tasks, like climbing stairs or even getting up from a chair or a sofa. This is why so many of us stay rooted at a spot- *getting up begins to hurt.* This, in turn, leads to inactivity, which is a further contributor to muscle loss. And we have a vicious cycle. The outcomes can range from an increased propensity to lose balance and fall, a loss of independence, and premature death.

So, is there any way to prevent this? Yes.

Exercise can prevent, hold off, and even reverse muscle loss and weakness. Physical activity can lead to better health, increase the turnover of protein, and restore the levels of signaling molecules involved in muscle function. These signaling molecules are gastro-transmitters like nitric oxide (NO), carbon monoxide (CO), and hydrogen sulfide (H2S), which play a critical role in regulating several physiological and pathological functions, including pathologies in connection with how we age (Butler-Browne et al., 2018).

Exercise can induce muscle cells to maintain youthful levels of gene transcription. Transcription is the preliminary stage in the expression of genes, where information from a gene is used to construct a functional product such as a protein. In 2002, a staff of the Mayo Clinic in Minnesota and his colleagues found that high-intensity aerobic training reversed numerous age-related differences, including restoration of mitochondrial protein levels, in muscle composition (Sreekumar et al., 2002).

Finally, exercise is also beneficial in inducing autophagy or cellular regeneration and restoration of myokine levels that decline with age. The myokines are necessary for the autocrine regulation of metabolism in human muscle tissues. Autocrine signaling is critical for cell growth.

Our muscles are the most abundant tissues we have. They account for 30 to 40% of our total body mass. Their functionality extends beyond keeping us mobile and helping us breathe. We also need muscles for glucose, lipid, and amino-acid homeostasis. In other words, our body stays in balance because of our muscles. It's never too late to begin training and taking care of your muscles.

The relationship between BMI and Your Mood

You may not know this, but your weight has subtle connections with the way you feel. So, if you are overweight and always feel tired, anxious, depressed, or frustrated, there is a reason for it.

It's been a common notion that overweight and obese people are naturally compulsive eaters and try to compensate for what they consider as deficiencies in their lives. Research suggests that with alarming numbers of overweight people, depressed people are likely to develop metabolic syndrome, which further contributes to excess visceral fat and weight gain. You may find that you rely on processed, junk food items that are cooked in harmful oils that do nothing good for your body to comfort yourself. This leads to lethargy and poor health, which in turn contributes further to depression and anxiety (*Effects of Obesity and Exercise: Is Obesity a Mental Health Issue? The Harvard Mental Health Letter Investigates*, 2014)

Obesity is linked with several diseases. This includes cardiovascular diseases, sleep apnea, lifestyle diseases like diabetes, and cancer. These diseases don't just affect us personally but can pose a significant economic drain on the country. There's an associated psychological burden linked to obesity. Studies have shown that 20-60% of people with obesity, particularly extreme obesity, suffer from some form of psychiatric illness (Sarwer & Polonsky, 2016).

A study conducted in 2003 aimed to analyze whether fitness levels, daily physical activity, and obesity can be signs for health-related quality of life and mood stability/instability in older persons.

The study revealed that aerobic fitness was associated with more desirable outcomes. The participants who had high aerobic fitness exhibited better tolerance of body pain, higher physical functioning, and vitality. Increased fatness contributes to increased anger, depression, and mood disturbance. The researchers concluded that even *small amounts of daily physical activity* within the purview of a normal lifestyle could lead to better health-related quality of mood and life (Stewart et al., 2003).

All you need to do is improve your fitness slightly and decrease your body fatness. Your body does not need you to climb a mountain. It just asks that you get up and move for a little bit in a whole day spanning 86,400 seconds. That's a lot of time, and all you need from it for better fitness is 420 seconds.

Health Concerns for Aged People

When it comes to maintaining your health, physical activity and a good diet can go a long way in helping you stay fit. If you do not take care of your health, you become susceptible to several age-related diseases. Some of these include:

- The CDC states that heart disease remains the leading killer of the aged population above 65. It accounted for 489,722 deaths in 2014 alone. Heart diseases are chronic and affect 37% of men and 26% of women above 65 years. As people age, they live with increased risk factors like high blood pressure and high cholesterol. This increases the risks of strokes or heart diseases. The only way to ameliorate this is with exercise, a good diet, and sufficient rest (Vann, 2016).

Scientists have increasingly studied and identified causes behind the aging of blood vessels and the heart and tried to understand how the aging, cardiovascular system leads to lifelong problems. The National Institute of Aging highlights the importance of regular physical activity as a shield against cardiovascular diseases. This is an essential factor in influencing the rate of aging of a healthy heart (*Heart Health and Aging*, 2018).

- Cancer is the second leading cause of death among aged people above 65. Around 413,885 deaths were reported in 2014 alone. The CDC reports that 28% of men and 21% of women are living with cancer. While one cannot always prevent it, measures can always be taken to ensure as much safety as possible.

  The University of Texas Cancer Center reports that staying active can help lower your risk of developing several cancers, including cancers of the breast, uterus, and colon. Exercise helps you maintain a healthy weight. Being obese increases the risk of cancers. Exercise regulates and controls your hormone levels. It also aids digestion, reducing the period within which harmful substances get to stay and wreak havoc in your colon (*Physical Activity*, 2021).

- Chronic respiratory diseases like *chronic obstructive pulmonary disease* (COPD) account for the third most common cause of mortality among people of and above 65. They were responsible for 124,693 deaths in 2014 (Vann, 2016). The American Lung Association recommends exercise for improved lung health. When we are active, our heart and lungs must work harder to supply additional oxygen to our working muscles. Exercise makes the heart and lungs stronger. So, with improved physical fitness, our bodies become efficient in pumping oxygen into the bloodstream and transporting it to our muscles.

Aerobic activities like walking, jumping rope, or jogging can give your heart and lungs the capacity to function efficiently. Muscle-strengthening activities like Pilates will build core strength, improve your posture, and tone your breathing muscles. Breathing exercises and yoga can help strengthen your diaphragm and equip your body to breathe deeper and more effectively (*Exercise and Lung Health*, 2020).

- According to the CDC, Alzheimer's disease accounted for 92,604 deaths of people over 65 in 2014. According to the Alzheimer's Research and Prevention Foundation in America, regular physical exercise can reduce your risk of Alzheimer's by up to 50%. It can also slow down cognitive disintegration in those who have started to develop symptoms.

Exercise protects against Alzheimer's and other variants of dementia by stimulating the brain's ability to preserve old connections and forge new ones.

- Osteoporosis is another health ailment that troubles us as we age. It is marked by the depletion of calcium in our bones, making them likely to fracture and break.

According to the National Osteoporosis Foundation, it is estimated that 54 million Americans over 50 are affected by low bone mass or osteoporosis. Regular exercise reduces the rate of bone loss and preserves bone tissues, therefore lowering the dangers and propensity of fractures. Exercising also reduces the risk of falling.

Since exercise improves your overall immunity, you are better protected against diseases that attack or weaken your health system. This includes influenza and pneumonia. Exercising doesn't just benefit one part of your body- it affects and changes your whole system for the better.

What's Holding You Back?

When it comes to exercise and physical activities, there is a marked reluctance among the aged population to pick up a daily activity. There are several reasons for this.

- Self-efficacy is a big issue when it comes to taking up an activity. We often feel unconfident when it comes to our abilities to perform and complete activities. As we grow older, we lose our confidence, mainly if the activity is a new one. This results from a perceived notion that we are not fit any longer, our bodies are not as competent, and we will make fools of ourselves. Contrarily, the more we sit in one place, the more this fear will develop. The only way to get rid of this fear is to get up and get moving.
- Another fear that results from the presumption that we are inherently unfit is a fear of injury. As we grow older, we become afraid that we may fall or get injured. Again, a sedentary lifestyle will only increase this conception because

we will grow more afraid as time passes. The only way to stop being afraid is to try the activity ourselves.

- Older adults are also embarrassed by the physical changes taking place in their bodies, including perceptions of appearance and self-worth. This causes problems since many may feel reluctant to step out and 'risk' being watched by others while exercising.

- Sitting around in one place also makes us develop inertia. We feel lazy and can't be bothered to expend energy on an activity. This causes a lack of determination and zero motivation to exercise.

- As older adults, we are also adjusting to more significant life changes. Many of us may be retiring, we may have children settled far away from home, loved ones passing, and frail family members who are older than us and need our care. These transitions can lead to feelings of depression, which take away from our desire to perform any exertions.

- Health problems like chronic illnesses, inflammation, joint pain, and disabilities become common issues that prevent older people from exercising. We become more afraid of further injury and hospitalization, pain, or simply assuming that we can't take up any more exercise. Again, this is a misconception because sitting around will only make our muscles stiffer.

- Older adults may be juggling a lot of work. They may be babysitting their grandchildren, volunteering, or being involved in other responsibilities, making them think that they can't be bothered to exercise.

- A section of the older population may not know how to exercise without instruction and advice. There's also a misconception that exercise has to be very hard and stressful to amount to something, and this misconception prevents people from picking up any activity.
- Some older adults think that lack of social and familial support is a significant barrier preventing them from exercising. It is human nature to want support when picking up something new, and it can be scary if there is none. If you have younger people in the family, try to involve them positively in your pick-up activities.
- Finally, many people also believe that exercise is expensive and requires a lot of fancy equipment, which is another myth. All you need is some minutes of each day and some space.

The ironic thing is that exercise can improve and reverse all these issues, and it can boost your spirits and make you fit and happy. So, don't let these myths keep you from becoming a better version of yourself. Consult a doctor before you begin to pick up an activity that is right for your age and fitness levels, and get started!

How To Use This Book

Let me take a minute to introduce myself. I have spent decades working with thousands of clients who belong to the age groups of and above 60. I've spent years researching and testing different fitness methods and techniques to find what sticks and what isn't sustainable. At this point, I have become extremely aware of how our bodies are tuned to different fitness activities, what works, and what doesn't.

Think of this question for a minute. Let's say you have spent years without control of your body and your faculties. You have lost your independence. What if you could reclaim it all? What if you could take back your balance, energy, and strength faster than you would have deemed possible? What if I gave you a field-tested perspective to exercise that will take no more than seven minutes of your time each day, and what if this resulted in visible positive changes in just seven days?

- This book will be your guide to learning a simple, scientific exercise plan that will take seven minutes, two times a day. It will provide consistent improvements in strength and mobility.
- We will cover simple bodyweight exercises which will target the very muscle groups whose functionality will help you stay active and independent while keeping your balance grounded so that you are no longer afraid of falling.
- We will discuss workouts that are home-based and do not require complicated, expensive equipment.
- You will learn the most important strategies for gaining the most from daily workouts.
- And finally, I will also talk about practical advice for your family and loved ones so that they can help and support you as you take up new activities.

The exercise programs in this book have been tested and verified by thousands of seniors and older adults who began from where you are now. It has helped them reclaim the very aspects of their lives that they felt were hopelessly out of control.

So, it doesn't matter if you start reading this book at 60 or 100, whether you are beginning at optimal fitness levels or zero, or if you are walking ten miles every day or struggling to get up from your couch. I will show you how to transform your body, and with it, your life, regardless of where you are beginning. What counts is what comes next and how much time and willingness you give to it.

Key Points

- Before we move on to the next chapter, here are some key points for you to remember!
- Most of the reluctance we face regarding exercise has to do with myths and misconceptions about our bodies and capabilities. The more active we are, the healthier we will become.
- Many age-related ailments like osteoporosis, arthritis, diabetes, cardiovascular issues, weak immunity, and other problems result from failing health. This directly connects with exercise, which can help us enhance and preserve our health and balance.
- The way your muscles age is directly related to exercise. If you don't exercise, your muscles become weaker.
- Lack of exercise can make your arteries stiffer, causing them to become brittle and tough over time. This can lead to high blood pressure and consequent problems like diabetes.
- There is a connection between exercise and your mood. Exercise keeps your BMI stable or lowers it to an ideal range,

which keeps you happy and healthy. Obese people are likelier to be frustrated and depressed.

- Finally, in this book, we will cover evidence-based exercise methods, tips, and tricks that will take a few minutes of your time every day. You will not need any expensive equipment, and you may reap results within seven days, provided you are dedicated and willing to introduce positive change in your life.

CHAPTER 2

The Benefits of Exercise for Older Adults above 60

By now, we know that there are various reasons we slow down and become more sedentary as we get older. It may be because of health issues, weight or pain issues, or fear of falling. Or, maybe you believe that exercise isn't for you. However, as you get older, maintaining an active lifestyle is more important than ever for your well-being.

Getting around will make you feel more energized, preserve your freedom, protect your spirit, and control sickness or pain symptoms, as well as your weight. Exercise is also beneficial to the mind, mood, and memory. It's never too late to find easy, fun ways to increase your physical activity, boost your mood and attitude, and reap the many physical and mental health benefits of exercise.

Physical activity has many advantages for people of all ages, but is it safe for seniors to exercise? According to the American Academy of Family Physicians, almost all older people will benefit from increased physical activity. Regular exercise, in reality, helps to avoid chronic disease, improves mood, and reduces the risk of injury. As we grow older, our bodies take longer to heal, but moderate physical exercise is beneficial to people of all ages and abilities. In reality, for the majority of people, the benefits of regular exercise far outweigh the risks. And older people with chronic illnesses may find healthy ways to exercise.

Physical activity and exercise can help older people in general and older people with health conditions. It can help improve quality of life, well-being, and physical function and reduce falls. A recent interview revealed that integrating multitasking exercise components with moderate physical activity positively impacted everyday lives, emphasizing the importance of physical, emotional, and social demands. Balance instruction can also be included in physical activity programs for older adults to help prevent falls. Exercise has also been shown to minimize the risk of falling by 21% (Langhammer et al., 2018).

Exercise and Physical Health

Let's take a moment to look at some great physical benefits of exercising!

- **Weight loss and maintenance**: Maintaining a healthy weight can be difficult when your metabolism slows as you get older. Regular exercise helps the body burn more calories by increasing your metabolism and building muscle mass. So, you can eat a healthy diet and still maintain your weight. As we get older, we find that we have to keep restricting our calories. This becomes an eventuality, but without exercise, our dietary options become more and more limited. By keeping our metabolism stable and functional, exercise allows us to have more options for food (Robinson et al., 2020).

- **Lowering your blood pressure:** Daily physical exercise strengthens the human heart. A stronger heart will pump blood far more quickly. The force on your arteries decreases as your heart works less to pump, reducing your blood pressure. Increasing your physical activity will lower your systolic blood pressure (the top number in a blood pressure reading) by 4 to 9 millimeters of mercury on average (mm Hg). That's comparable to the effects of certain blood pressure drugs. Exercise can be sufficient for certain people to minimize the need for blood pressure medicine.

  If your blood pressure is within a healthy range (less than 120/80 mm Hg), exercise will help keep it from increasing as you get older. Exercise also aids in the maintenance of a healthy weight. You must continue to exercise regularly to keep your blood pressure low. Daily exercise can take anywhere between one to three months to affect your blood pressure. However, for the effects to last, you have to maintain a daily activity schedule (*Exercise: A Drug-Free Approach to Lowering High Blood Pressure*, 2019)

- **Decrease the potential consequences of sickness and chronic disease**: Exercise boosts immune and digestive function, lowers blood pressure and increases bone density, and reduces the risk of Alzheimer's disease, type 2 diabetes, obesity, cardiovascular disease, osteoarthritis, as well as some cancers in people.

- **Help you deal with asthma:** People with asthma will benefit from exercise in a variety of ways. This includes increasing lung capacity, improving lung and heart blood flow, increasing endurance and stamina, reducing airway inflammation, and improving overall lung health. In addition to prescription drugs, exercise will help you manage your asthma symptoms (Nunez, 2020).

- **Exercise can help ease back pain:** Exercising the back decreases stiffness by keeping the ligaments and tendons' connective fibers flexible. Improved back mobility helps to keep the connective fibers from tearing under tension, which helps to prevent damage and back pain.

- **Improve your agility, endurance, and coordination**: Exercise strengthens your stamina, flexibility, and posture, which can help with your balance and coordination while also lowering your risk of falling. Strength training can also assist with the effects of long-term illnesses like arthritis.

- **Increase longevity**: Were you aware that exercise has the potential to add years to your life? Researchers at The Journal of American Medical Association (a peer-reviewed journal) put this theory to the test. The research looks into the connection between long-term mortality and different levels of *cardiorespiratory fitness* (CRF). CRF is a metric that measures how effectively the heart and lungs pump blood and oxygen across the body during extended periods of exercise.

The higher your degree of CRF, the more suited you are. CRF can be increased by both regular and intensive exercise.

Participants ranged in age from 18 to over 80, with an average age of 53. Fitness was linked to living longer, as found in previous studies (Ahmed, 2019). Interestingly, the researchers also discovered a connection between CRF and survival rates: the higher one's fitness level, the better one's chances of surviving. This was particularly noticeable in the elderly and those with high blood pressure. And the survival value continued to rise steadily (Ahmed, 2019).

Exercise and Mental Health

Did you know that exercise has visible mental-health benefits as well? If done correctly, it can become the basis of a happy, fulfilled life.

- **Exercise helps you sleep better**: As you grow older, getting enough sleep becomes more important for your overall health. Regular exercise will assist you in falling asleep more quickly, sleeping more comfortably, and waking up feeling more energized and refreshed. From archaea to humans, the circadian rhythm is an evolutionarily conserved system. Circadian rhythm modulates biological activity to arrange an optimal timing for each process in response to day-night shifts in the environment on Earth. Circadian rhythm and exercise have a strong relationship, whereby the latter significantly impacts upon and restores balance in the former (Wang, 2017).

- **Exercise boosts your self-esteem:** Exercise is a great stress reliever, and the endorphins released during activities help alleviate feelings of grief, depression, and anxiety. Being active and feeling good can also make you feel better about yourself, and if you struggle with body image issues, it is a great way to stabilize your feelings and be proud of yourself.

- **Exercise aids brain function:** Exercise doesn't just help with physical balance; it also aids us in developing a mind-body connection. It can help with time management and innovation. It also acts as a shield against memory loss, cognitive impairment, and dementia. Being involved in regular activities can also help to delay the development of brain-related ailments like Alzheimer's.

- **Exercise can cure depression:** There's a scientific explanation as to why exercise can act as a cure against depression. Exercising triggers a biochemical loop with various health benefits, including reducing blood pressure, enhancing sleep, and preventing heart disease and diabetes. Endorphins, the body's feel-good chemicals, are released during high-intensity exercise, resulting in the "runner's *high*" that joggers experience. However, for most of us, the real benefit comes from sustained low-intensity exercise. The release of proteins known as neurotrophic or growth factors, which allow nerve cells to expand and form new connections, is triggered by this type of action. You will feel better as the brain function improves (*Exercise Is an All-Natural Treatment to Fight Depression*, 2021).

Neuroscientists have discovered that the hippocampus, a brain region that helps control mood, is smaller in people who are depressed. Exercise helps alleviate stress by promoting nerve cell development in the hippocampus and enhancing nerve cell relations (*Exercise Is an All-Natural Treatment to Fight Depression*, 2021).

Now that we have read about the different advantages of physical exercise, we can pause for a minute and think of how the benefits will apply to us. Each of these will change your life for the better, only if you find the strength in you to overcome your misgivings.

Of course, you will feel restrained by several personal and physical misgivings as you age. What's important is developing a regular physical routine. This doesn't mean anything too hard or stressful. Strenuous exercises or visits to the gym aren't needed to reap the benefits of exercise. Adding more movement and action to your life, even in small amounts, can have a significant impact (Robinson, 2020). Over time when older people lose their ability to do things independently, inactivity is mostly to blame rather than age. Lack of physical activity can lead to further medical visits, emergency room visits, and increased medication usage for several illnesses.

Key Points

Before we move on, let's do a quick review of what we read in this chapter!

- Daily exercise is a great way to keep your body in shape and your organs healthy. Contrary to misconceptions, it is an essential way to stay fit as you age.

- Exercise has many physical benefits. It can help you lose weight and maintain a steady weight so that you don't have to compromise on your diet all the time.
- Exercise can help reduce or maintain blood pressure so that you don't become a victim of hypertension.
- Asthmatic patients can reap the benefits from exercise and increase lung capacity.
- Back pain can be alleviated with specific exercise schedules.
- Exercise improves agility, balance, and endurance.
- Exercise can have the effect of increasing your lifespan.
- Other than physical benefits, exercise can also boost your mental health.
- Your body has a natural circadian rhythm. Disturbance of this rhythm can cause a lot of imbalance in your sleep cycle. Exercise helps maintain this rhythm and benefits your sleep.
- Exercise helps in brain function and increases your cognitive capacities. It helps against the early onset of neurodegenerative disorders like Alzheimer's.
- Exercise is a great way to boost self-esteem and allows you to feel confident about yourself.
- You can bring intimacy back into your life with a healthy exercise schedule.
- Finally, exercise contributes to the release of endorphins, which boost your happiness and cure depression.

CHAPTER 3

Common Misconceptions about Fitness at age 60 and over

Several misconceptions about exercise keep us from being more physically active and retaining our strength as we grow older. In these cases, we must note that mindset is everything, and the majority of these myths are tricks being played by our minds and excuses that we tell ourselves to justify not doing what we know we should do.

Myths about exercise and older adults include, but are not confined to, claims that older people are too vulnerable to do resistance training for fear of damaging their already fragile bones. This is due to the mentality that older people can only get marginal health benefits from physical activity. However, rebutting common fitness myths and re-educating older adults on proper exercise techniques may significantly promote frequent and healthy physical activity participation (Sell & Frierman, 2010).

Many of us believe that we don't have the energy or endurance we need for exercise. Contrarily, the more involved you are, the greater your tolerance for physical activity and the more you can do during the day. Your activity tolerance decreases as you become less active, and according to research, participation in sports and exercise has shown to increase overall physical activity and energy levels. Maintaining an active lifestyle will help you lower your resting heart rate, improve blood flow, and even boost your metabolic rate. Exercise improves energy efficiency by increasing blood flow, supplying more nutrients and oxygen to muscles.

Let me share a small story with you. Many years ago, when I first started working in the physiotherapy department, I found that many of the patients were in their 60s. Some would be able to run marathons, and others would arrive in a wheelchair at the clinic. The distinction was in the mentality of trying to take care of yourself. The patients who were confined to wheelchairs came with the inherent mentality that they could not fend for themselves, even though they could get better with effort. They felt depressed and spent most of their time sitting around watching television. The physically active group, however, engaged in activities regardless of their age and abilities. As a group, they were happier and healthier.

Common Myths and Misconceptions about Old Age and Exercise

There are several myths and misconceptions linked with old age, and I will highlight some of the key myths that prevent older people from starting physical activities.

Myth One: With age, you lose your capability to exercise.

Contrarily, the more involved you are, the greater your tolerance for physical activity and the more you can do during the day. Your activity tolerance decreases when you stop engaging in any form of physical activity. Subjects who exercised for 20 minutes three days a week for six weeks experienced a 65 percent reduction in fatigue, according to a University of Georgia report (Puetz et al., 2008).

According to research, participation in sports and exercise has increased overall physical activity and energy levels. Maintaining an active lifestyle will help you lower your resting heart rate, raise your blood pressure, and even boost your metabolic rate.

Myth Two: People above 60 are too old to exercise.

Fauja Singh is the oldest surviving marathon runner, having completed his last race at the age of 101 in 2013. He has shown that age is only a number and has no bearing on your ability to exercise. In 2015, 49% of runners who completed a marathon in the United States were in the "masters" category, meaning they were 40 years old or older. In addition, home fitness routines were studied in 200 people aged 60 and up in a randomized controlled study. After the project, improvements in balance and impairment ratings were assessed. There were no adverse health effects reported by any of the participants (Evans, 2017).

According to Dr. Thomas Boyden, MS, program director of *preventive cardiology* at *SHMG Cardiovascular Medicine in Grand Rapids, Michigan*, anyone (regardless of age) can stimulate their heart and lungs to raise their heart and breathing rate. Stimulation of the cardiovascular and respiratory systems lowers the risk of cardiovascular diseases, such as heart attacks and strokes, and the risk of cancer (Citroner, 2019).

Myth Three: What's the point of exercise if I'm growing old anyway?

Physical exercise makes you look and feel younger while also allowing you to remain independent for longer. Exercise reduces the risk of neurological disorders like Alzheimer's and dementia and heart disease, diabetes, some cancers, high blood pressure, and obesity. The effects of exercise on one's mood can be just as strong at 70 or 80 as when they were 20 or 30. This myth is more of complacency, a human desire to remain stuck where we are because any form of change, no matter how positive the effects, takes some effort. If you feel resistant, remind yourself of the good things that will follow once you pick up any form of physical activity.

Myth Four: Exercise increases my risk of falling and damaging my bones.

Contrary to this myth, regular exercise reduces bone loss and improves balance, lowering the risk of falling by increasing strength and endurance. Osteoporosis is a condition that causes brittle, frail, and easily broken bones in over 200 million people around the world.

Osteoporosis affects 30% of postmenopausal women, and one out of every six women is prone to breaking their hip once in their lifetime. There are ways to reinforce your bones as you get older. The majority of these interventions would also boost physical health and length of life. And all of these interventions require you to get up and get moving (*5 Ways to Strengthen Older Bones*, 2021).

For instance, several studies have marked increases in bone mineral density, bone strength, and bone size were observed in older men and women who engaged in weight-bearing exercise (Klentrou et al., 2007).

Myth Five: I've been an athlete once. I don't have what it takes to do it all over again.

With age, overall strength and efficiency levels will inevitably decrease due to changes in hormones, physiology, metabolism, bone density, body composition, and muscle mass. But that doesn't rule out the possibility of gaining a sense of accomplishment or improving your health through physical activity. The key is to set realistic lifestyle goals for your age group. Also, keep in mind that a sedentary lifestyle has a much more significant impact on physical performance than biological aging.

The good news indicates that the age-related decrease in maximal heart rate is lower in athletes than in non-athletes. Older people who engage in intensive exercise training are likely to reap the same benefits as their younger counterparts.

In addition, several other variables can work in your favor. Older athletes, for example, are more likely to practice 'intelligently' – that is, to use a more scientific approach to training, such as a structured and oriented training schedule (rather than just putting in the miles) and to use dietary techniques to improve success and recovery. Older athletes are generally better at recognizing their responses to training and tailoring a curriculum to their needs rather than blindly pursuing a "*one size fits all*" strategy (Hamilton, 2021).

Myth Six: Oh, this is too hard! I'm too old for exercise!

You need to remember that it is never too late to start exercising and improving your fitness! Adults who become physically and mentally active later in life also display more significant changes than their younger counterparts. If you've never exercised before or haven't done so in a long time, you won't suffer from the same sports injuries as many daily exercisers do later in life. In other words, you won't have to worry about the fear of pain from older injuries resurfacing. Start with simple routines and work your way up (Robinson et al., 2020).

According to Dr. Richard J. Hodes, director of the NIH *National Institute on Aging*, it is important to get started and stay active regardless of your activity levels in your youth. We must understand that people need to be self-sufficient for as long as possible. Older people can maintain their physical function by exercising more and having more physical activity in their daily life, which is important for doing the things they want to do.

Myth Seven: I'm disabled, so exercise is an absolute no for me!

Being challenged brings its own set of issues. You face unique challenges if you are confined to a chair. However, you can increase your range of motion, enhance muscle tone and endurance, and encourage cardiovascular health by lifting light weights, stretching, and doing chair aerobics, chair yoga, and chair tai chi. Many swimming pools are accessible to wheelchair users, and adaptive fitness programs for wheelchair sports like basketball are also available. According to the 2008 *Physical Activity Guidelines*, people with disabilities can follow the same guidelines as healthy adults or do as much as possible to prevent becoming inactive (Rosenberg et al., 2011).

A famous study on this topic is the *Lifestyle Interventions and Independence for Elders (LIFE)* study. The LIFE study looked at the probability of long-term physical activity in improving a significant mobility challenge. The study considered that if any participant could not walk 400 meters, they had a mobility disability. The participants were anywhere between 70-89 years of age. They were divided into two groups, one that received exercise and one that received health education but no exercise. By the sixth month of this study, the participants in the exercise group could perform an extra forty minutes a week of medium-intensity exercise, and they could continue this after 12 and 24 months (*Study Reveals Performing Light Physical Activity Prevents Major Mobility Disability among Elderly*, 2020).

| Myth Eight: I'm far too weak to exercise.

Moving around will help you relieve pain while also improving your strength and self-esteem. Many older people discover that daily exercise slows and strengthens the deterioration of strength and stamina that comes with age. The goal is to take it slowly and build up and add more activities as you get stronger.

Several studies of stable older people conducted in the 1970s found that resilience, endurance, and flexibility decline dramatically after 55. According to the *Framingham Disability Report*, 62% of women aged 75 to 85 had trouble bending or bowing down, 66% couldn't carry more than 10 pounds, and 42% couldn't stand for more than 15 minutes. These declines were once thought to be an unavoidable part of growing older. However, *Harvard and Tufts* researchers published a seminal study in 1994 found that many functional losses could be reversed, particularly in the frailest and oldest women (*Exercise after Age 70*, 2019).

For ten weeks, 100 nursing-home occupants ranging in age from 72 to 98 completed resistance exercises three times a week. The exercise group could lift substantially more weight, climb more stairs, and walk faster and further at the end of the study than their sedentary peers, who tended to lose strength and muscle mass. Other researchers have also confirmed the importance of exercise for the elderly and disabled communities. The collective opinion is that the more active you are, the healthier your life will be (*Exercise after Age 70*, 2019).

More Myths Holding Older Adults Back from Exercising

Many people believe they are too out of shape, sick, exhausted, or just plain old to exercise because they are out of shape, sick, tired, or just plain old. They are mistaken. Regardless of your age, movement is *always good.* Let's look at some reasons why older adults are so reluctant to exercise.

- Some of us accept that physical and mental decline is just an inevitability of growing old. According to Chhanda Dutta, Ph.D. and chief of the *Clinical Gerontology Branch* at the *National Institute on Aging*, there's a powerful misconception that growing older equals being frail and incapacitated. However, the reality is quite different. There are people in their 70s, 80s, and 90s who are running marathons and competing in bodybuilding competitions. According to Alicia I. Arbaje, MD, MPH, and assistant professor of *Geriatrics and Gerontology* at *Johns Hopkins University School of Medicine* in Baltimore, many of the symptoms we associate with old age are simply symptoms of inactivity, not age (Griffin, 2021).

- Exercise benefits your well-being in more ways than one. It can also help with memory and dementia prevention. Exercise can also assist you in maintaining your freedom and way of life. You'll be able to keep doing the things you love when you get older if you remain strong and agile. You'll also be less likely to need assistance.

- Some of us have this fear that exercising will give us heart attacks. This is only possible if you choose an activity that is beyond your capacity. To prevent that, you need to consult with a physician and come up with a wholesome routine. As a matter of fact, you are much more at risk of cardiovascular diseases without exercise.

- As we age, and particularly if we age in a sedentary setting, our joints get weaker, and many develop arthritis. This makes us more reluctant when it comes to taking up any physical activity. Exercising can seem too painful if you have arthritis. Exercising has been shown to help with arthritis pain, which may seem counterintuitive. According to a report, people over 60 with knee arthritis who exercised more had less pain and improved joint function (Griffin, 2021).

- One of the common and most harmful delusions we feed ourselves with is that we don't have time. Experts suggest a minimum of 150 minutes of aerobic exercise per week. When we read it like this, it does sound like a lot. But, it adds up to a little more than 20 minutes per day. Furthermore, you are not required to complete it all at once. It's possible to divide it up. You can take a ten-minute walk in the morning and a fifteen-minute jog in the evening when the weather is cool- and you're done for the day! Also, we will discuss routines that will take only seven minutes of your time, which is something that all of you can contribute to your well-being.

- Finally, we have some misgivings that result from a lack of understanding. Some of us may think exercise is too expensive and gyms are for young people. That is not true. A world of activities exists out there which requires nothing but for you to move your body. Gyms are for everyone, but if you feel

40

uncomfortable, you can always work out at home. As a matter of fact, that is what we cover in this book. And, while some of us may think that exercise is tedious, it's not. It is a great way to get fit and enjoy our lives!

Is Age the only factor to blame for poor health?

You are never too old to take up a form of physical activity. It is simply essential that you educate yourself on where and how to begin. For instance, in a study, 130 senior citizens aged 60 and up (average age 67 years) with eight years of schooling took part in Greek traditional dance sessions for 32 weeks. The sessions lasted 75 minutes each and were conducted twice a week. Initially, moderately intense dances from all over Greece were selected. During the show, they were able to experiment with higher-intensity dances. At the start and end of the intervention, the participants' physical health was assessed using scientific tools. The findings established that their physical health had greatly improved (Douka et al., 2019).

To conclude, the most significant barrier to establishing and continuing a healthy routine that will uplift and strengthen us exists in our minds. We have to internalize the belief that we are capable of substantial, significant change. Think of how much your body has already done for you! It has borne you through these many years of your existence, and it deserves some nourishment and care. Any physical activity you engage in becomes an act of you giving back to your body. Embrace it with positivity.

Key Points

Before we move on, here are some key points to summarize what we read in this chapter!

- As older adults, we often give in to misconceptions and myths that keep us from engaging in physical activity.
- Many of us think that we are too old to take up anything new. Physical activity is a great way to protect our bodies as we age.
- Some of us have been athletes and sporty when we were younger, and we think we can't do it again. But, if we focus our minds on it, we can build new routines specific to our age.
- There's a misconception that people above 60 are too old to exercise. Did you know that the world's oldest marathon runner completed his last race at 101 years of age? You are never too old to take care of your health.
- We think that exercise increases our chances of falling and breaking bones. Contrarily, exercise is a great way to prevent osteoporosis and help us regain our balance and bone density.
- Mobility disability is not a barrier to exercise; as a matter of fact, the latter can help you stay healthy and positive. Exercise is also a great way to protect our bodies from degenerating because of chronic health conditions.
- You are not too weak for exercise. The more stationary you stay, the weaker you get- so this myth is counterintuitive.
- Exercise protects you from neurodegenerative disorders like dementia, allowing you to remain independent and in control of your identity.

- If you choose a proper routine, you do not need to be afraid of issues like heart attacks, which can only happen if you pick up something far too difficult. Nobody expects you to become a sprinter at 70. Proper consultation with a physician and knowing what works for your body will help immensely, and finally,

- Never convince yourself that you don't have the time for exercise. It takes 7-10 minutes a day. You can find that time for bettering your health.

CHAPTER 4

How to Exercise at Home with Minimum Equipment

Although lifting weights is beneficial to all, older adults will benefit even more if they work for a stronger, healthier body. A healthy body can help you prevent accidents, falls, discomfort, and other problems that come with aging. If you don't do enough to preserve your muscle mass when you get older, you can eventually lose it. You will live longer if you maintain or add muscle, and you will have a better quality of life. We'll talk about how you can get involved in physical activity in this chapter. The exercises are designed to improve total-body strength while also enhancing balance, stability, and flexibility. Let us now look at different exercises to help you get and stay fit!

Introduction to Stretching

As we age, daily tasks such as getting out of a chair and getting into and out of bed become difficult. These restrictions are often caused by a loss of muscle strength and flexibility. The ability of muscles and tendons to lengthen and stretch in response to movement and enable a joint to move across its range of motion is called flexibility. To retain flexibility, it is essential to integrate a successful stretching program into your daily routine (Pletcher, 2019).

Stretches for the neck, arms, back, hips, and legs will help you retain your flexibility as you age, keeping you limber for all life has to bring. Stretching allows for more joint mobility and enhances posture. It also aids in the relaxation of muscle tension and soreness and the prevention of injury. Finally, it can boost circulation, muscle strength, and balance coordination.

Before we discuss some key stretches, here are some things you should remember when you do stretching exercises.

- When you stretch, take a deep breath and slowly exhale in between each stretch.

- Hold each stretch for 30 seconds to allow your muscles to relax.
- Don't bounce when stretching because it raises the risk of injury.
- Stretch only until you feel the tension build up in the muscle, not until it hurts. Our goal is to warm your body, not cause distress to it.
- Warm-up for 5 to 10 minutes before stretching by moving about, such as going for a stroll.

Calf Stretches

The calf is found at the back of the lower leg, just below the knee. It is made up of two muscles: the gastrocnemius and soleus. Muscle tightness and cramping are typical in the gastrocnemius muscle. These may occur as a result of muscle exhaustion or a lack of stretching.

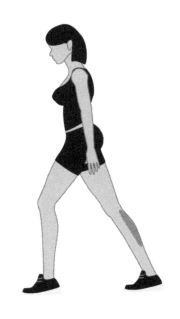

Stretching regularly will increase a person's range of motion, allowing muscles to lengthen and contract more vigorously during exercise. Stretching can help avoid cramping and tightness by improving muscle contraction. Calf muscle stretches for seniors, such as the one shown below, are important for maintaining leg flexibility. Seniors can easily execute this exercise by leaning against a wall or a chair.

Performing the Stretch

Step 1: Stand at arm's length from a wall, a heavy chair, or a piece of durable exercise equipment.

Step 2: Place your palms flat against the wall or grip the piece of equipment.

Step 3: If you cannot use any of these, simply stand at balance as best as you can, one foot in front of the other, the knee of the front leg slightly bent.

Step 4: Position one leg back, knee straight, and heel flat on the floor.

Step 5: Slowly bend your front knee while moving your hips forward until you experience a calf stretch.

Step 6: Maintain this posture for 30 to 60 seconds.

Step 7: Switch leg positions and repeat for the opposite leg (Tucker, 2018).

Things to remember

- Begin with the basic calf stretch. Do this for at least a week until you progress to the other stretches.
- Every time you attempt a stretch, feel your muscles relaxing and easing up.
- Each of you may be at varying levels of flexibility. Some of you may find it easier to stretch; some may feel a persistent tightness. Be patient with yourself.
- Finally, and most importantly, consult a health professional before you attempt any of these stretches.

Shoulder Stretches

Stretching your shoulders is a great way to release tension that has built up in them and reduce pain in your arms' joints. There are unique stretches and exercises that can be particularly helpful if you have shoulder tightness, healing from an injury, or want to increase the strength of your shoulder muscles. Incorporating shoulder-specific exercises and stretches into your overall workout routine can help you improve your shoulder mobility and flexibility. These movements can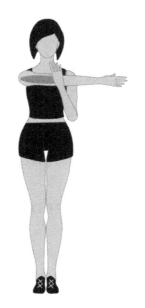
also help you develop shoulder strength, improve shoulder function, and avoid injury (Lindberg, 2020).

Performing the Stretch

The most basic shoulder stretch would require you to

Step 1: Stand tall, your legs together, arms relaxed. Keep your eyes straight ahead.

Step 2: Bring your left hand across your right shoulder in one clean vertical movement.

Step 3: Using your right hand, grasp your left shoulder and tug until you feel a stretch. Keep your breathing even.

Step 4: Release, return to your starting position and repeat with the right hand.

Things to remember

- Stop immediately if you feel any pain. If there is a sharp nudge or twitch that hurts you when you do these exercises, do not proceed.
- Breathe evenly so that you can relieve stress and tension in your shoulders. Breathing will also help you hold a post for longer.
- Start with baby steps. If you are new to exercise or to shoulder exercises, don't push too hard too soon. Start with some simple stretches and add more as your balance develops.
- Before you do any of the exercises, consult with your doctor or physical therapist. They will help you identify any irregularities that you may need to address (Lindberg, 2020).

Triceps Stretch

Triceps stretches increase endurance, muscle length, and range of motion. Furthermore, they can help avoid tight muscles, loosen connective tissue, and increase circulation while requiring little or no equipment. Triceps stretches are arm exercises that target the large muscles in the back of your upper arms. These muscles are responsible for elbow extension and shoulder stabilization.

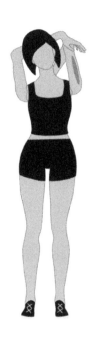

The triceps collaborate with the biceps to execute the majority of heavy forearm movements. They're important muscles for building upper-body strength, which is particularly important as you get older. Stretching the triceps improves flexibility and can help avoid injuries (Cronkleton, 2019). We will discuss a basic overhead triceps stretch.

Triceps Stretch: Performing the Stretch

Step 1: Lift your shoulders toward your head, then lower and back.

Step 2: Extend your right arm to the ceiling, then bend at the elbow to pull your right palm toward the center of your back, with your middle finger resting along your spine.

Step 3: Gently bring your elbow in toward the middle and down with your left hand.

Step 4: Hold this particular stretch for 30 seconds and repeat three or four times on each hand.

Things to remember

- Stretching the triceps can help to alleviate pain and distress. However, you should avoid doing these stretches if you are in severe pain or have questions about your bones or joints.
- If you've recently injured yourself, wait until you're nearly healed before beginning the stretches.
- If you experience some discomfort during or after these stretches, stop immediately.
- Build up slowly, particularly if you aren't usually physically active or have neck, shoulder, or arm issues (Booth, 2020).

Quadriceps Stretch

The quadriceps help stretch the knees and are used in daily tasks such as getting out of a chair, walking, and ascending stairs. We depend on our quadriceps to perform several daily tasks, and if we spend a lot of time sitting, they can become tight.

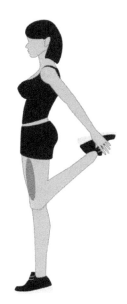

In turn, though stretching the quadriceps appears to be a relatively simple way to ensure muscle tightness does not occur in this region, the quadriceps can be challenging to stretch. This is because you have to lift your leg and stand on one leg, which can be difficult if you have mobility problems with your knee or hip or balance issues.

Muscle tension in the quadriceps can cause back and knee pain, general tightness, and decreased mobility, but a few minutes of stretching can save you from a weekend of agony on the couch. Exercises to improve flexibility for seniors and the elderly, such as quadriceps stretches, are important for maintaining hip and leg range of motion (Shrift, 2006).

Basic Standing Quadriceps Stretch: Performing the Stretch

Step 1: Standing tall and keeping on to a solid surface to maintain your stability.

Step 2: Bring your foot up to your buttocks while reaching out and grasping your foot.

Step 3: Make sure your knees are in line with each other and that you are standing tall.

Step 4: Hold for the specified amount of time before repeating on the opposite leg.

Things to remember

As always, judge yourself before you begin the exercise.

- Do you feel fine? Does any muscle hurt when it shouldn't? Are you relaxed?
- If you have any injury in the area you are stretching, consult your doctor before beginning anything.
- Try to stop arching your lower back too far.
- If your hamstring cramps, pause, wait for it to uncramp and then resume.

Neck Stretch

When the head and shoulders sag forward due to poor posture, specific muscles in the chest and neck will shorten and tighten over time, perpetuating the poor posture and causing neck pain. The area above your shoulders is often tense, mainly if you sit at a desk all day (with poor posture) or are constantly looking down at your phone screen. Neck pain, according to science, may feel like a "kink," discomfort, or extreme pain. This pain may spread to your shoulders, upper back, or arms, or it may cause headaches and arm numbness, tingling, or weakness (Mansour, 2019).

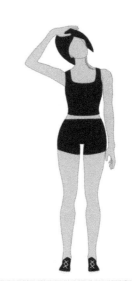

Neck Stretch: Performing the Exercise

Step 1: Maintain a straight back and a square head over your shoulders.

Step 2: With your left hand, gently touch the left side of your head and tilt it to the left. Go as deep as you can, and you should feel a stretch on the right side of your neck.

Step 3: Hold the stretch for 15-30 seconds before slowly turning your head forward.

Step 4: Repeat on the other side.

Things to remember

- A neck stretch is amazing because of its functionality. You can do it anywhere, including sitting in a chair in front of your computer.
- Make sure you do not feel any pain when stretching your neck.
- As always, if you feel uncomfortable, it is best to consult with a health professional for signs of latent injuries before you begin.

Leg Stretch

Many people have tight calf muscles. We also start to get a little tighter as we age, and our muscles lose a little water content and extensibility. It is extremely important to stretch out the leg muscles to keep them relaxed and malleable. The more relaxed the muscles are, the greater your functionality.

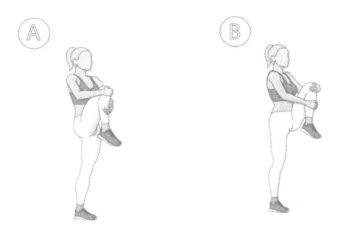

Leg Stretch: Performing the Exercise

Step 1: Stand with your feet shoulder-width apart, back straight, eyes in front of you.

Step 2: Gently raise your right leg, with your knee bent, to a comfortable level for you. As you get more efficient, practice raising your knee to your chest. You may need to hold on to something like a chair to keep your balance.

Step 3: Hold your knee with the palms of your hands for 15 seconds. Feel the stretch.

Step 4: Lower your right leg. Pause for ten seconds, and repeat with your left leg.

Things to Remember

- Don't begin with the intent to reach your knee to your chest on the first day. Begin slowly and build your strength.
- If something feels wrong, consult with a health professional.

Hamstring Stretch

For adults and the elderly, hamstring stretching is a vital part of lower back and leg endurance. When we get older, our lower body begins to stiffen and lose freedom of motion.

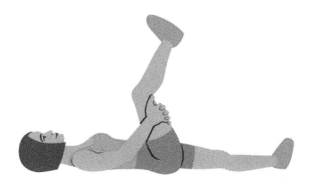

We begin to realize this gradually. It hurts to wear our shoes and socks. Getting up from a chair is painful. When we try to reach down, our hamstrings feel tight and hurt. This loss of range of motion can affect our physical mobility. To prevent these things, stretching your hamstrings is of utmost importance.

Hamstring Stretch: Performing the Stretch

Step 1: Lie flat on a surface, buttocks down, feet flat on the field, legs bent.

Step 2: Bring your right leg to your chest slowly.

Step 3: Extend the leg while maintaining a slight bend in the knee. To deepen the stretch, use a yoga harness or rope; don't pull too hard.

Step 4: Hold for 10 seconds and gradually increase to 30 seconds.

Step 5: Repeat on the other knee. Then, for a total of two or three times, replicate this stretch with each leg.

Things to Remember

- It is important to keep your hamstring muscles loose. Tight hamstrings are more likely to strain or break. If you have hamstring pain, you should see a doctor before trying to cure it at home.

- You can keep your hamstrings loose by doing a variety of workouts and stretches. Warming up your muscles before stretching is a smart idea. Take a stroll or engage in some other exercise to fire up your body.

- Never stretch while you are in agony, and never attempt to push a stretch. When stretching, keep a regular breathing pattern.

- Have hamstring stretches in the routine at least two to three times a week.

Inner Thigh Stretch

You use the muscles of your inner thigh and your groins more than you realize. These muscles play an important role in keeping you upright, steady, and going safely every time you walk, move, or bend. The adductors are the inner thigh muscles. They are composed of five distinct muscles. These muscles are connected to the pelvic (hip) bone and the femur (upper leg bone). Your adductors are essential for stabilizing your hips, knees, low back, and heart, in addition to assisting you in moving safely. Stretching these muscles will help you remain mobile late into your life.

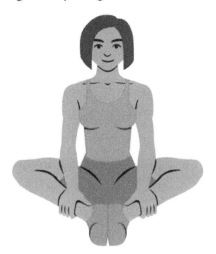

Inner Thigh Stretch: Performing the Exercise

Step 1: Sit on the ground with your feet joined together in front of you. Allow your knees to fold out to the sides.

Step 2: Place your hands on your feet and draw your heels toward you.

Step 3: Maintain a straight back and engaged abs as you relax your knees and inch down to the floor. You'll feel some pressure on your groin muscles.

Step 4: Breathe deeply and keep this pose for 15 to 30 seconds.

Step 5: Repeat three times more. For a deeper stretch, bring your feet closer to your crotch.

Things to remember

- Don't bounce or perform sudden, jerking motions. Muscles may be injured or torn by sudden, jerky, or bouncy movements.
- Begin slowly. Don't try to do too much too soon. Start with a few stretches and gradually increase the number as your versatility improves.
- Don't forget to take deep breaths. Breathing helps alleviate stress and tension in your muscles and allows you to maintain a stretch for more extended periods.
- Don't go above what you're happy with. Any discomfort is natural, but you should not experience pain while stretching. If you feel a sharp pain, stop immediately.
- You should also see a doctor if you have pain that worsens when you walk or sit or have difficulty moving your legs.

Introduction To Bodyweight Training

Bodyweight training (or strength training exercises that do not include free weights or machines) came in second place on *The American College of Sports Medicine's* list of the top 20 global fitness trends for 2014. Some people may be wary of a workout that does not require costly equipment or heavyweights, but research shows that bodyweight workouts boost stamina, endurance, and power and can burn a lot of calories if done correctly (*The Benefits of Bodyweight Training*, 2021).

Bodyweight training is relatively simple compared to complex exercises that require a lot of instruction and expensive equipment. As we grow older, these exercises help us develop balance and coordination. If we focus on our bodies, which is what bodyweight training needs us to do, we need our total concentration on the exercises we are doing. This not only improves physical strength but acts upon and strengthens our mind-body connection.

Before we go into different examples of bodyweight training, here are some things to keep in mind.

- Take five to ten minutes, warm up, and cool down. Walking is a great way to warm up, and stretching is a great way to cool down.

- Concentrate on your form rather than weight. Align the body correctly and move through each exercise smoothly. Injuries and slow progress can result from poor form.

- Working at the proper pace allows you to maintain stability rather than sacrificing strength gains due to momentum. For example, count to three while lowering a weight, hold it, and then count to three while bringing it back to its starting position.

- During your workouts, pay attention to your breathing. Exhale as you lift, push, or pull against resistance; inhale as you let go.

- Maintain muscle resistance by gradually increasing weight or resistance. The appropriate weight for you depends on the workout.

- Maintain your routine — working out all of your main muscles twice or three times a week is perfect. You can do a full-body strength workout twice or three times per week, or you can divide your strength workout into upper- and lower-body components. In that case, make sure you do each part at least twice a week.

- Allow your muscles to rest. Small tears in muscle tissue are caused by strength training. These tears aren't harmful, but they serve a purpose: they help muscles grow stronger as the tears bind together. Allow 48 hours for your muscles to heal before your next strength training session.

We will now discuss several bodyweight exercises. We will also talk about the difficulty levels of each exercise so that you have options to choose from. Consult a professional before you begin any of these exercises.

Hip Raise Exercise

Your glutes are one of the biggest and most efficient muscles in your body. However, sitting for long periods at a desk will cause these muscles to forget how to function. You'll be weaker in almost any lower-body workout as a result of this. Furthermore, poor glutes can lead to a forward tilt of the pelvis. This not only places more strain on your lower back, but it also forces your lower abdomen outward, making your stomach protrude—even though you're not overweight. On the other hand, the hip lift allows you to reactivate your glutes and develop muscle all over. Your glutes are also one of your body's top calorie burners because they're such a large muscle group. As a result, the hip raise will help you burn more fat in the long run.

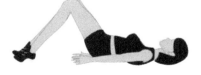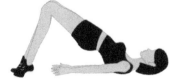

Particulars

Difficulty Level: Easy

Equipment Needed: None

Repetitions: 20 times for three sets with 10-second breaks between each.

Hip Raises: Performing the Exercise

Step 1 (Starting Position): Lie down on your back, knees bent, and feet flat on the ground.

Step 2: Make a 45-degree angle with your arms out to your sides.

Step 3: Squeeze your glutes tightly and brace your abdomen.

Step 4: Then, lift your hips to form a straight line from your shoulders to your knees.

Step 5: Pause for five seconds while keeping your core braced and squeezing your glutes, then return to the starting spot.

Step 6: Repeat.

Things to Remember

- Your hips and torso should shift in unison. As a result, the arch in your lower back should stay the same from beginning to end. This way, you're focusing on your glutes rather than your lower back and hamstrings.
- This exercise should come first in your routine, before any other lower-body exercises. This will help unlock your glutes and enable you to squat, deadlift, and lunge with heavier weights.

Dumbbell Curl Exercise

Dumbbell curls are a great exercise for strengthening the arm muscles. Seniors should try not to skip them while working out. The dumbbell curl is a common movement that targets the biceps located on the front of your upper arms. This exercise's success stems in part from the many benefits it provides. While dumbbell curls are primarily aimed at the biceps, the exercise also works with various other muscles. The brachialis and brachioradialis are two of the many muscles employed by the bicep curl. The former is found under your bicep, while the latter is in your forearm.

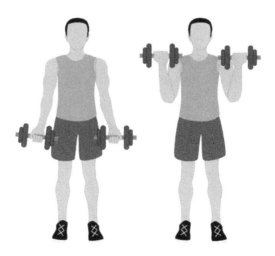

Dumbbell curls are necessary because the muscles and movements that are conditioned by this exercise are highly functional. Every day, you flex your arm at the elbow joint countless times, from picking up a suitcase and lifting a beverage or simply raising your hand to yawn. The bicep curl is necessary because it can help with these daily tasks.

Particulars

Difficulty Level: Easy

Equipment Needed: A pair of dumbbells, weighing four pounds each. You can increase the weight as you become more efficient, but do not start with more than four pounds in each hand.

Repetition: 5 times on each hand.

Performing the Exercise

Step 1 (Starting Position): Start by standing erect with your feet hip-width apart. Keep the abdominal muscles taut.

Step 2: Hold a dumbbell in each of your hands. Allow your arms to hang down by your sides, palms facing forward.

Step 3: Bend at the elbow and raise the weights so that the dumbbells approach your shoulders while keeping your upper arms stable and shoulders relaxed. Keep your elbows pulled in tight to your ribs. When lifting, exhale.

Step 4: Return your hands to their original positions. Don't bounce or swing your arms.

Step 5: Perform five curls on each hand. Increase to 10 after a week, and proceed depending on your level of comfort.

Things to Remember

Concentrate on correct posture rather than speed. Lift the weights in a smooth movement, taking the same amount of time to lower as you did to raise it.

When you are doing the curl, keep your elbows in the same position. They should stay tight to the body's side, with only the lower arm moving. You are probably lifting too much weight if you find your elbows shifting away from your torso or drifting in front or behind the body.

When performing the dumbbell curl, do not use your shoulders or torso to swing the weights up. This can result in a swinging, twisting, or heaving movement.

Maintain a long, upright spine as well as a tight heart. Maintain a relaxed posture and keep your shoulders from moving forward to initiate the movement. If this happens, use lighter weights or reduce the number of repetitions.

90-90 Crunch Exercise

If you want better abs and core strength, you can do 90-90 crunches. It stimulates the rectus abdominis muscle. Since crunch exercises require you to be in complete control of your body, they can help you concentrate on your workout routine. This exercise will also help you gain muscle strength and flexibility.

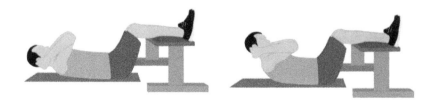

Particulars

Difficulty Level: Easy
Equipment Needed: A bench or a chair (should be a medium height).
Repetitions: 10 times.

Performing the Exercise

Step 1 (Starting Position): Keep a chair or a bench in front of your legs. The chair or bench should be near your feet so that you can raise your legs to it.

Step 2: Gently lift both your legs to the chair or the bench. Your legs should be straight and above your hips, not going too high or too low. Keep your hands behind your head.

Step 3: Raise your head to your knees till you feel a crunch in your abdomen. Hold for one second, and return to the starting position. Don't rush it.

Step 4: Repeat ten times.

Things to Remember

- Involve your core as best as you can. This is a core exercise, so the muscles should strain, and it should feel like you are using them.
- Raise your upper body from your abdomen.
- Keep your legs evenly placed throughout. Don't move them or bounce them because this will release tension.

- If ten repetitions become too much, begin with five and increase as you become more comfortable.

Dumbbell Shoulder Shrug Exercise

If you work at a desk, you probably spend a large portion of your day with your neck bent forward with your shoulders slouching. This pose can strain your neck and shoulder muscles over time. Shoulder shrugs are a common exercise for strengthening your shoulder muscles as well as your upper arms.

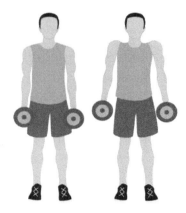

The *trapezius* muscles are the primary muscles targeted by shoulder shrugs. These muscles can be found on either side of your body. They are in control of the movement of your shoulder blades, as well as the upper back and neck.

You will find it easier to maintain correct posture if these muscles are improved by exercise. A solid *trapezius* muscle draws your shoulders back and aids in stabilizing your neck and upper back.

Particulars

Difficulty Level: Easy.

Equipment Needed: Two dumbbells, four pounds each.

Repetitions: Total 15 times.

Performing the Exercise

Step 1 (Starting Position): Begin in a standing position with your feet flat on the floor. Your feet should be shoulder-width apart.

Step 2: Maintain your arms at your sides with one dumbbell in each hand.

Step 3: Bend your knees slightly to align with (but do not extend past) your toes. Maintain a straight neck and chin by keeping the chin up.

Step 4: Bring your shoulders as far up into your ears as you can when inhaling. Slowly perform the movement so that you can feel the resistance of your muscles.

Step 5: Lower the shoulders and exhale before repeating the action. Do a total of fifteen repetitions.

Things to Remember

Shoulder shrugs are simple exercises. There aren't many steps to take or directions to obey. However, there are some safety precautions to follow if you attempt this exercise.

- When doing a shoulder shrug, never roll your head.

- Raise your shoulders carefully before lowering them back down in the same vertical direction.
- If you get tired before fifteen repetitions, stop and rest. Do only as many as you can take. Increase as your endurance goes up.

Dumbbell Overhead Shoulder Press Exercise

If you want to improve your back mobility, it's important to keep your upper body muscles in good shape. These muscles assist you in performing daily tasks such as putting dishes up high in a cabinet or placing things overhead on a shelf. Perfo-rming the overhead press, also known as a shoulder press, is a great way to keep the upper body in shape in your overall workout routine.

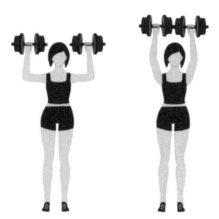

There are some advantages of incorporating the overhead press into your workout routine. Overhead pressing can improve shoulder muscle strength and size, increase the triceps muscles' strength and scale, and help you build core muscle strength, tone your transverse abdominal muscles, lower back, and stabilize your spine.

Particulars

Difficulty Level: Easy

Equipment Needed: Two dumbbells, four pounds each.

Repetitions: Perform this exercise a total of 15 times in 1 repetition. Do two repetitions with a 30-second break in between.

Performing the Exercise

Step 1 (Starting Position): Maintain a straight back and stand tall.

Step 2: Raise your hands from your elbows. Hold a dumbbell in each hand. Pause at the shoulders. This will be the point from which you begin the exercise. The thumbs should be on the inside, and the knuckles should be facing up.

Step 3: Exhale as you raise the weights above your head in a controlled motion. Once your hands are fully extended above your head, stop.

Step 4: When inhaling, return the dumbbells to the shoulders.

Things to Remember

- For this exercise, always choose a weight that you are comfortable with.

- Do not bounce or swing your arms; you may harm yourself. Make the motions steadily, and if you find them difficult, stop and come back when you are ready.
- Don't let your arms move back and forth. They should move straight up and then back to your shoulders.
- When you are returning to a neutral position, do so slowly to avoid any injuries.

Leg Raise Exercise

This exercise works on lower back muscles, buttocks, hips, and thighs. Seniors achieve greater balance by improving these areas. It increases overall body strength and endurance, which is a significant advantage for someone who spends several hours sitting at a desk. Leg raises are a strength training exercise that will help you develop core strength while lying down.

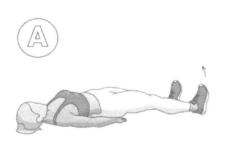 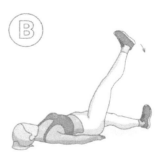

Particulars

Difficulty Level: Easy
Equipment needed: None

Repetitions: Perform this exercise a total of 15 times in 1 repetition. Do two repetitions with a 30-second break in between.

Performing the Exercise

Step 1 (Starting Position): Lie on your back with your hands at your sides.

Step 2: Hold your knees up and your feet on the mat/floor.

Step 3: Use your core muscles to lift your legs straight up in the air.

Step 4: Lower your legs halfway or all the way, depending on your comfort level, and then raise them back up.

Step 5: Breathe in as you lower your legs and exhale as you raise them.

Things to Remember

- Do not lift your shoulders when doing the exercises because this will focus on the wrong muscles.
- Do not apply undue pressure on your chest.
- Do not arch your back when you bring the legs down; your back and spine should always be in a neutral position.
- As always, begin with 15 reps, and you can gradually increase this to 25 as you become more experienced. If you feel uncomfortable, take a break between two repetitions.

Triceps Dips Exercise

The triceps dip exercise is an excellent bodyweight exercise for developing arm and shoulder strength. This basic exercise can be performed almost anywhere and comes in various variations to suit your fitness level. It can be used as part of an upper-body power exercise. One of the most powerful exercises for stimulating the triceps muscles in your upper arm is the triceps dip. You'll also stimulate your core because you'll be holding your hips off the ground rather than lying on the floor or sitting.

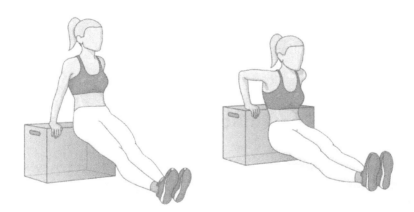

Particulars

Difficulty Level: Easy

Equipment Needed: A stable chair or a bench.

Repetitions: Perform this exercise a total of 15 times in 1 repetition. Do two repetitions with a 30-second break in between.

Performing the Exercise

Step 1 (Starting Position): Sit on the edge of a chair or a bench, and grip the edge next to your hips.

Step 2: Your legs should be extended in front of you, and your feet kept hip-width apart, with your toes touching the ground. Maintain a straight face and a high jaw.

Step 3: Lift your body with your hands and move forward just far enough so that your behind clears the edge of the chair.

Step 4: Lower your body using your triceps till your elbows are bent between 45 and 90 degrees.

Step 5: Repeat by slowly pushing yourself back up to the starting spot. Maintain control of the movement across its range of motion. Do not bounce or jump.

Things to Remember

- Maintain a relaxed posture with your shoulders down and away from your face. Your shoulders should not be raised.
- Take note of the pressure on your shoulders. If you start to feel a lot of pressure, don't go any lower. Otherwise, you risk injuring your shoulder.
- At the top of the movement, do not lock your elbows. Maintaining stress on the triceps by keeping them slightly loose.
- When you lean forward, you are working your chest muscles rather than your triceps. Keep a straight line with no forward-leaning movement.

Donkey Kick Exercise

Donkey kicks are excellent for increased stability as well as toning. They work on your gluteus maximus, which is the largest of your three gluteal muscles. Since your whole body must stay relaxed as your leg lifts, they also work your heart and shoulder muscles. This exercise stretches the hip in the opposite direction than how we keep it while we sit, and it also helps to offset those sedentary hours in a chair. Both of these aid in the improvement of posture and the prevention of hip and spine injuries.

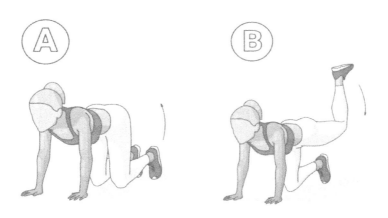

Particulars

Difficulty Level: Easy

Equipment Needed: None

Repetitions: 20 times on each leg.

Performing the Exercise

Step 1 (Starting Position): Get down on all fours, with your knees at hip's distance from each other. Keep your hands under your shoulder. Your neck and spine should be neutral.

Step 2: Balance and engage your core, and start lifting your right leg. Keep your knee bent, foot flat, and hinged at the hip.

Step 3: Using your glute, press the foot towards the ceiling and squeeze it at the top. Make sure that your pelvis and the working hip are pointed to the ground.

Step 4: Return to the initial position without bouncing. Go at an even pace.

Step 5: Complete 15 repetitions on each leg and repeat the whole movement twice.

Things to Remember

- The donkey kick is a simple exercise, and you have to be focused on your form to do it correctly.
- Aim at isolating your glutes, and make sure that you are comfortable.
- Stay in control of your movements, and if you cannot do 15 repetitions, begin with 10.

Bird Dog Exercise

The bird dog is the main exercise that works on improving your stability, helps you keep your spine neutral, and eases lower back inflammation and pain. It balances and strengthens your core, back muscles, and hips. It also helps you develop good posture and enhances your range of movement. It is excellent for preventing injuries, spine alignment, and helping you recover from back spasms.

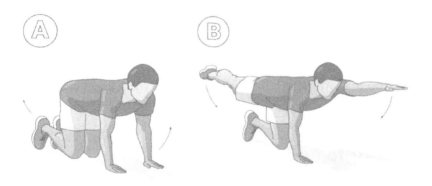

Particulars

Difficulty Level: Easy.

Equipment Needed: Exercise Mat.

Repetitions: 20 times.

Performing the Exercise

Step 1 (Starting Position): Go down on all fours on the exercise mat.

Step 2: Position your knees beneath your hips and keep your hands below your shoulders.

Step 3: Keep your spine neutral and your core muscles engaged.

Step 4: Draw the blades of your shoulders together.

Step 5: Lift your right arm and left leg, all the while keeping your hips and shoulders aligned to the floor.

Step 6: Push your chin to your chest and look down to the floor. Hold this position for 15 seconds.

Step 7: Ease back into the starting position.

Step 8: Now, raise your left arm and your right leg, and hold for 15 seconds. This becomes one complete set.

Step 9: Repeat the whole movement 20 times.

Things to Remember

- Your breathing should be aligned and even.
- Do not rotate your pelvis or bounce from your hips.
- Don't lift your leg higher than necessary because this will make your spine curve beyond its natural stance.
- Don't let your back sag.
- Don't let your chest sink to the floor; keep it as neutral as possible.
- Keep your shoulder blades drawn back and away from your ears.
- Move like you are in control of the movement.

Single-Leg Deadlift Exercise

The single-leg deadlift increases hip strength and power and enables the hip and leg muscles to serve as stabilizers. When you stand on one knee, you use the same muscles for balance and stability that are usually used for force development. Balance can be improved by forcing the body to develop equilibrium on one leg. It is also excellent for building strength.

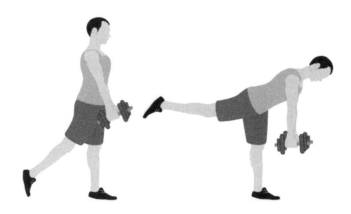

Particulars

Difficulty Level: Intermediate
Equipment Needed: A pair of dumbbells, four pounds each.
Repetitions: Do 20 reps total, and increase this to 30 as you develop stronger muscles.

Performing the Exercise

Step 1 (Starting Position): Begin by standing with your feet parallel and hip-width apart. Hold two dumbbells in front of you with your hands down.

Step 2: Lean forward in your hips, transferring your weight to one leg as the other leg engages and begins to stretch straight behind you.

Step 3: Lift your extended leg and lean forward until your body forms a "T" shape. Your arms should be straight down, gripping the weight.

Step 4: Maintain a slight bending of your standing leg. Return to the starting place by slowly bringing in your extended leg. Repeat with your opposite leg.

Things to Remember

- Throughout the lift, the back must stay neutral. If you round or flex your back, you risk injuring it.
- The front knee will bend, but it will not shift too far forward. Keep in mind that we are deadlifting, not squatting.
- The shoulders and hips remain parallel to one another and to the surface. Don't let your back leg externally rotate, and don't let your working hip fall or rise above parallel.
- Make sure the knee does not collapse inward or outward.
- Maintain a focus of around 3-6 feet in front of you to help keep your head in line and aid in balance.

- As your torso moves forward, keep your shoulders connected to your spine.

Two-arm Bent Over Row Exercise

Weight-training exercises allow you to improve your strength while also improving your health. Strength training advantages include improved muscle mass and bone health by creating resistance for muscles to resolve. Specific movements, such as bent-over rows, target several muscle classes, resulting in increased physical strength and endurance. When combined with cardio training and good nutrition, the result is a leaner, more toned physique.

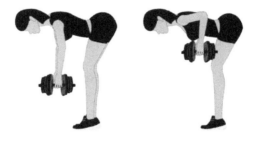

Free weights, weight machines, body weight, and gravity can all be used to provide resistance. Bent-over rows use free weights and gravity to provide movement resistance. Another benefit of using dumbbells is the ability to train each side separately, which aids in identifying and correcting left-to-right imbalances. It also aids in overall muscle stabilization.

86

Particulars

Difficulty Level: Intermediate.

Equipment needed: A pair of dumbbells, each weighing four pounds.

Repetitions: Perform this exercise a total of 15 times in 1 repetition. Do two repetitions with a 30-second break in between.

Performing the Exercise

Step 1 (Starting Position): Stand with your feet shoulder-width apart, holding a dumbbell in each hand with a neutral (hammer) grip.

Step 2: Flex your leg muscles until your body is horizontal or close to horizontal, maintaining a natural curvature of your spine.

Step 3: Let the dumbbells hang down by your arms and extend your shoulders downward.

Step 4: Exhale as you raise the dumbbells to the sides of your waist, keeping your elbows tight to your neck.

Step 5: Squeeze the back muscles and hold for a count of two.

Step 6: Lower the dumbbells to the starting position while inhaling and extending the shoulders downward.

Step 7: Repeat.

Things to Remember

- Maintain a normal curvature of the spine by keeping the neck level and head up.
- Pull with your elbows, not your biceps.

- Keeping your torso horizontal (or nearly so) and your elbows tucked in will ensure that you activate the correct muscles.
- Start slowly to give your lower back time to adjust. Remember never to bounce.

Dumbbell Bent-over Row Exercise

Most people don't give their back much thought until it fails them, and they're forced to lie in pain on a wooden floor for hours. Internal shoulder rotation causes tight pecs and a sore neck. This sometimes results in lower back fatigue, causing pain and discomfort at best and threatening severe injury at worst. The issue is only exacerbated if you put more stress on the chest and shoulders with endless pressing exercises. Put more emphasis on your back training. The bent-over row should take a step forward.

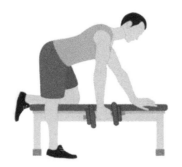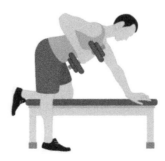

The bent-over row benefits your back muscles the most because as they strengthen, your posture improves, so you don't sag as much. The two-arm bent-over dumbbell row works several muscles in the upper and middle back. That includes the *trapezius, infraspinatus, rhomboids, latissimus dorsi, teres major, and teres minor*, and *posterior*

deltoid. The *pectoralis major* of the chest and the *brachialis* of the upper arm is also employed. Your shoulder rotators are in use. This is a compound, practical exercise, and you can use this motion during the day while picking up items. Knowing how to align your back and brace your abs correctly will help you avoid strain.

Particulars

Difficulty Level: Intermediate

Equipment Needed: A pair of dumbbells, four pounds each, and a bench or chair.

Repetitions: Perform this exercise a total of 15 times in 1 repetition. Do two repetitions with a 30-second break in between.

Performing the Exercise

Step 1 (Starting Position): Raise your left leg on the exercise bench (your bench should be at a thigh-high level) and hold the far left side of the bench with your left hand.

Step 2: Bend over so that your upper body is parallel with the ground.

Step 3: Reach down with your right hand and pick up a dumbbell. Keep your grip neutral. Your palm should face you.

Step 4: Hold the dumbbell with an extended right arm, keeping your back straight.

Step 5: Bring the dumbbell to your chest. Make sure that you lift it with your shoulder and back muscles, not your arm muscles. Keep your chest even and breathe.

Step 6: At the top, squeeze your shoulder and the muscles of your back. Gently lower the dumbbell until your right hand is fully extended below. Repeat 15 times on the right hand, and switch.

Things to Remember

- Throughout the exercise, you must maintain a straight back and square shoulders.
- You must not lift the weights above the shoulder line.
- Your body should be lowered and aligned to a maximum of 45 degrees. Further bending over can cause back strain, particularly if you are lifting heavier weights.
- Do not unnecessarily bend the wrist up, down, or perform any swinging motions.
- After you establish your stance and pick up the weights, your legs and hips remain stationary during this exercise. Do not attempt to squat.
- Do not attempt to lift heavy weights with this exercise unless you are an accomplished lifter who has confidence in your coordination, shoulder joints, and back.
- This is an intermediate-level exercise, so only do this if you are at a comfortable place with weight-lifting.

Side Plank Exercise

The side plank is one of the most straightforward exercises you can perform to engage the layers of muscles along the sides of your abdomen. These are your oblique muscles, and they help you rotate and bend and protect your spine. Side planks work on strengthening your shoulders, hips, and core, so you get three benefits for the work. They protect you from back injuries and don't put pressure on your lower back area. They strengthen your balance and help you build your focus on holding yourself in place. So, they engage both your mind and your body.

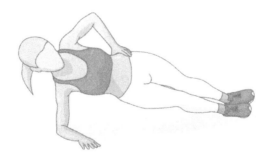

Particulars

Difficulty Level: Intermediate

Equipment Needed: None

Repetitions/ Time Needed: Hold in plank position for 40 seconds on each side. Build on this till you can hold for a minute on each side.

Performing the Exercise

Step 1 (Starting Position): Lie on your right hand, legs straight, feet stacked on top of each other.

Step 2: Place your right elbow under your right shoulder, forearm pointed away from you, and hand balled into a fist. Your pinkie finger should be in contact with the ground.

Step 3: Breathe out and brace your abdominal muscles while keeping your neck neutral.

Step 4: Lift your hips off the mat so that your weight is supported by your elbow and your right foot. From your knees to your shoulders, your body should be in a straight line.

Step 5: Maintain this posture for the remainder of the exercise. Aim for 40 seconds, and you can increase this depending on your fitness level.

Step 6: Repeat all the steps on the other side.

Things to Remember

- You shouldn't perform this exercise if you have any shoulder, arm, or abdominal pain. If you feel any pain during the exercise, stop immediately.
- If you have trouble holding the side plank, try performing the exercise on your knees. You can try it on your feet once you have built more strength.
- Avoid rotating your body.
- Don't let your hips sag. If 40 seconds feels like too much, do fifteen instead, but with good form.

Single-Leg Lift Exercise

When crossing your legs or walking up a flight of stairs, you normally lead with the same leg. Repeatedly working on one side of the body results in a strength imbalance, which, if severe enough, can lead to chronic pain and injury. This is because an imbalance causes some muscles to overcompensate and function harder than they should, increasing the risk of overworking and injuring them.

Single-leg movements, also known as unilateral exercises, will help you correct an imbalance. Acting with one side of the body at a time prevents the other side from taking over, so you're essentially pushing each leg to do the work without any assistance. That's also why they're perfect for testing and improving your equilibrium.

A single leg lift is a calisthenics and Pilates exercise that mainly targets the abs while occasionally targeting the hip flexors and lower back to a lesser extent. It imitates many of the gestures we make in our daily lives. After all, we don't always keep both feet on the ground as we walk, or run or engage in physical activities like playing sports. This form of exercise will improve your overall functionality since it closely resembles how you move your body in real life.

Particulars

Difficulty Level: Intermediate.

Equipment needed: None.

Time on each leg: 10 seconds, increased by 10 seconds every five days.

Repetitions: 5 times on each leg.

Performing the Exercise

Step 1 (**Starting Position**): Choose a clean space, and lie down with your legs and back flat on the floor or a mat.

Step 2: Rest your arms in a neutral position on your sides.

Step 3: Maintaining your legs straight, lift your right leg with your feet up until it points straight in the air. Hold for 10 seconds.

Step 4: Gently lower your right leg down. Don't rush it, don't bounce.

Step 5: Repeat with the other leg.

Step 6: Do this five times on each leg.

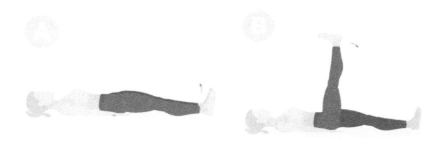

Things to remember

- Be in control of your movements. This is very important because if you jump or bounce, you will injure yourself.
- If 10 seconds seems like too much on the first day, hold your leg in balance for 5 seconds. As you get comfortable, increase this duration.

- Keep your arms neutral. They should not be engaging in this exercise because this will shift the balance from your legs to your arms, which we do not want.

Dumbbell Floor Chest Press Exercise

While it works with a short range of motion, the dumbbell floor press offers an excellent means of triceps isolation. It also strengthens other parts of the upper body, particularly the chest and shoulders. It improves core power. The floor press is a shoulder-friendly exercise because of its neutral grip and partial range of motion. Partially extending the arm often puts more stress on the triceps muscles, which help with maximum utilization and strength-building.

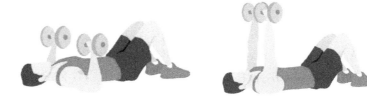

Particulars

Difficulty Level: Intermediate
Equipment Needed: A pair of dumbbells, four pounds each.
Repetitions: Repeat this 30 times for two sets.

Performing the Exercise

Step 1 (Starting Position): Keep your dumbbells on the floor, with enough distance between them for you to lie down on your back. Start by bending your knees and bring your feet up to your buttocks.

Step 2: Raise the dumbbells above your head, keeping your shoulders planted to the floor.

Step 3: Allow your upper arms to come down to your chest. Take a breath and squeeze your chest muscles.

Step 4: Repeat this motion 30 times.

Things to Remember

- Your arms must be in a straight position, don't bounce or jerk them.
- Don't rush the movements. Go slow and in control.
- Keep your eyes overhead as you perform the exercise and your breathing even.

Forward Lunge Exercise

Lunges are a common strength training exercise for people who want to improve, shape, and condition their bodies and improve overall health fitness. This resistance exercise is common because it can strengthen your back, hips, and legs while enhancing mobility and stability. Lunges are excellent for building your balance and body function.

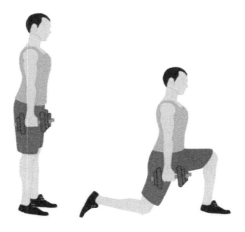

Since you function on each side of the body individually, lunges are a lower-body unilateral exercise. Single-leg movements engage your stabilizing muscles, which helps you improve balance, coordination, and stability. Working on one leg at a time makes your body less secure, requiring your spine and heart to work harder to maintain equilibrium.

Lunges are safer for recovery than bilateral exercises because they can fix imbalances and misalignments in the body and make it more symmetrical. If you have a weaker or more versatile hand, spend extra time focusing on it to overcompensate or overuse the dominant side.

Particulars

Difficulty Level: Intermediate
Equipment Needed: None
Repetitions: 5 on each leg.

Performing the Exercise

Step 1 (Starting Position): Stand tall with your feet at a hip's distance from each other. Feel a tension building up in your core- this means that your core is getting engaged.

Step 2: Take a big step in front of you with your right leg. Do this movement with your heel so that the weight of your body is resting on the heel and not the tip of your foot.

Step 3: Gently shift your full body weight on the right leg. At this point, the left leg will only be supporting you.

Step 4: Lower your body until your right leg becomes parallel with the floor, and the right shin is vertical. Your knee can bend forward a little, which is fine, *but make sure it does not go ahead of your toe. This is very important.*

Step 5: Press into the right heel and move back up to the starting position. When doing this, keep your balance intact. Don't bounce or jump back into it.

Step 6: Repeat on the other side.

Things to Remember

- Avoid bending at the hips and allowing your upper body to slump, as this will place more pressure on your knee.
- When lunging, you should take a step forward so that your front foot does not pop off the floor. If you take too shallow a move, your knee will travel forward past your foot, causing undue stress and strain on the knee.
- Avoid putting your front foot directly in line with your back foot. This has a negative impact on your stability and balance.

Dumbbell Split Squat

Split Squats are great for lower body stability because they are a powered stretch. When you lower yourself into the movement, the weight of your body and whatever implements you're carrying puts a greater tension on your muscles. Furthermore, the muscles must work hard to push back out of that deep range. When you stretch in this manner, you teach your body to have power in the deep range of movement you need. Split squats are also excellent for avoiding strength imbalances between the left and right legs.

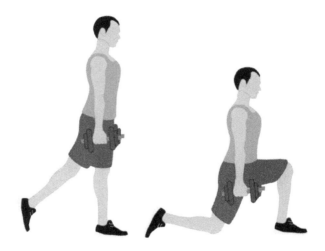

Particulars

Difficulty Level: Intermediate

Equipment Needed: A pair of dumbbells, four pounds each.

Repetition: 5 times on each hand.

Performing the Exercise

Step 1 (Starting Position): Stand straight, holding dumbbells by your side. Lunge forward with your right leg, keeping the left leg behind.

Step 2: To improve the range of motion, place the left foot behind as steadily as possible.

Step 3: Return to the starting point with the heel of your right foot.

Step 4: Repeat with the left leg. Once you return to the starting position with the left heel, one repetition is complete.

Step 5: Repeat until the required number of repetitions has been reached.

Things to Remember

- Focus on taking a slightly narrower split stance and driving up through the ball of the foot if you want to target the quads during the split squat.
- Always keep your stance neutral, don't jump or bounce.
- Don't feel like you have to be perfectly upright when doing the movement. On the opposite, you should lean slightly forward to keep the lumbar spine neutral.

Dumbbell Side Bend Exercise

Dumbbell side bends mainly target the Oblique muscles that run from the rib cage to the hip bone. Building up the oblique muscles can help stabilize the core/trunk/torso area and improve your balance and posture. One of the most common exercises for targeting the oblique muscles is the dumbbell side bent. It is essential to have sufficient oblique strength to maintain proper posture and protect the spine.

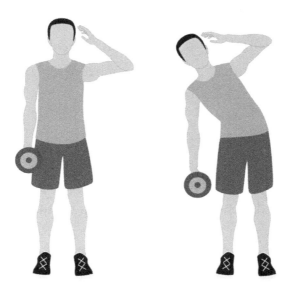

Particulars

Difficulty Level: Intermediate

Equipment Needed: One 8 pound dumbbell.

Repetitions: 5 times on each side.

Performing the Exercise

Step 1 (Starting Position): Hold a dumbbell in your right hand, palm facing in, and stand straight.

Step 2: Maintain a shoulder-width stance with your feet firmly planted on the concrete.

Step 3: Bend over to the right as far as you can while keeping your back straight and your eyes forward, then back up.

Step 4: Repeat 5 times, then repeat the whole movement on the left.

Things to Remember

- Always keep your back straight, your eyes forward, and just bend at the waist.
- Focus on stretching and contracting the oblique muscles (down the side of your body).
- Maintain a steady grip on the dumbbell, and never swing your hands in random motions.
- As a variation, this exercise can also be done sitting on the end of a bench.

Fire Hydrant Exercise

Bodyweight exercises such as fire hydrants, also known as quadruped hip abductions, primarily target the gluteus maximus, but some variants target the heart as well. Fire hydrants will help you sculpt your glutes, relieve back pain, and reduce your risk of injury if you do them regularly. They'll even help you shift your hips better. This can help to relieve back pain, improve posture, and make daily movement easier.

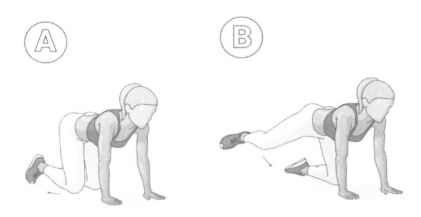

Particulars

Difficulty Level: Intermediate

Equipment Needed: None

Repetitions: Do ten repetitions on the left leg three times, and repeat with the right leg.

Performing the Exercise

Step 1 (Starting Position): Begin by going down on your knees and hands. Position your shoulders above your hands and keep your hips above your knees. Tighten your abdomen and keep your eyes lowered.

Step 2: Lift your leg and push it away from your torso, maintaining a 45-degree angle. Keep the knee balanced at 90 degrees.

Step 3: Lower the lifted leg to the starting position. This is one repetition. Do ten of these for three sets on each leg.

Things to Remember

- Maintain a balanced core and pelvis. The only thing that can move is your hip. Otherwise, the hips and glutes will be engaged.
- Guide your foot toward the opposite wall when you raise your knee. This will facilitate proper hip rotation.

Air Squats Exercise

Air squats are an excellent way to practice the proper technique of squatting. They also aid in the development of a strong foundation of strength and balance in your lower body. They specifically target your calves, hamstrings, quadriceps, and glutes, assisting you in preserving muscle mass in these areas. Air squats also engage your core because balance is needed.

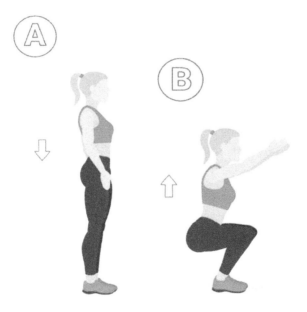

Particulars

Difficulty Level: Intermediate
Equipment Needed: None

Repetitions: Do 20 repetitions when you start; build to 40 repetitions.

Performing the Exercise

Step 1 (Starting Position): Maintain your feet at shoulder's distance from each other, toes pointing straight out.

Step 2: Move your arms forward.

Step 3: Squat and move your hips down and back. Descend your hips slightly lower than your knees.

Step 4: Gently return to starting position, and repeat.

Things to Remember

- Make sure your knees do not extend beyond the tips of your toes.
- Your back should not curve inward.
- Dropping your shoulders forward is not a good idea. The only part of your body that moves should be your lower body.
- Keep your gaze fixed on the wall in front of you. Your chest will remain elevated as a result of this, which is necessary for this exercise.

Crunches Exercise

Abdominal crunches are used to tone the body's core muscles. The exercise will help you strengthen your core muscles, improve your posture, and increase your muscle mobility and flexibility. Although these exercises will not wholly burn fat from the body, they will increase muscle mass and improve the body's ability to burn fat efficiently. In addition, the muscle density is improved.

Since they help strengthen your abdominal wall muscles, abdominal crunches are a highly effective approach to maintaining and improving balance. They play a critical role in posture improvement. You will notice that if your posture is optimized, you will perform more effectively in everyday tasks, but you will also avoid lower back pain and back muscle injuries.

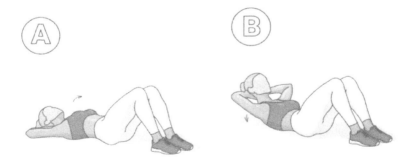

Particulars

Difficulty Level: Intermediate
Equipment Needed: None

Repetitions: Begin by doing 20 repetitions. As you get stronger, increase to 40.

Performing the Exercise

Step 1 (Starting Position): Lie flat on your back, feet planted on the ground. Place your arms and hands behind your neck, and bend your knees.

Step 2: Breath in with your abs. You should feel a contraction.

Step 3: Breathe out and lift your upper body slightly. Your neck and head should be relaxed.

Step 4: Inhale and go back to your starting posture.

Step 5: Repeat this 20 times, maintain an even pace.

Things to Remember

- Raise your upper body with the help of your core, not your neck or your back. If you use these, you compromise the exercise and risk injury.
- Control your movements and move slowly. You may think that moving quickly will work better, but contrarily, they won't affect the right muscles.
- Try placing your hands behind your neck once you have the proper form practiced. If you do it before that, you can injure your neck.

Single-Leg Bridge Exercise

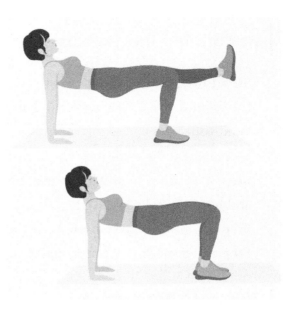

Bridge exercises are a great way of keeping your lower body active. They work the muscles at the back of your body and are powerful tools for activating your glutes. They strengthen hip mobility and your lower back, and because they are low-impact, they are suitable for anyone with hip issues. You use your glute muscles every day, whether you are going for a walk or picking up a laundry basket. These exercises will ensure you do these daily activities without pain and discomfort. They also increase core stability and improve your lower back, and this can improve your postural health.

Particulars

Difficulty Level: Advanced

Equipment Needed: None

Repetitions: 20 times, to begin with, increase to 40 as you grow stronger.

Performing the Exercise

Step 1 (Starting Position): Tighten the muscles in your abs and buttocks. Go down on the ground with your chest pointed out. You should be flat on your back.

Step 2: Raise your hips and hands to form a straight line between your knees and shoulders. Balance your hands on your palms, and keep the palms facing inward.

Step 3: Try to pull your belly button back toward your spine by squeezing your core.

Step 4: Slowly raise and extend one leg while maintaining a raised and level pelvis. Pause and hold for five seconds.

Step 5: Keeping your knees bent, return to the starting position.

Step 6: Repeat the whole process with the other leg. Do this 20 times, ten repetitions with each leg.

Things to Remember

- Never allow your back to arch- remember that the exercise must be performed from your glutes and not the back muscles.
- You should maintain a straight line from your shoulders to your knee. Do not rotate or sag your hips. If this happens, plant your leg back to the floor and do double leg bridges.

Walking Lunges Exercise

The static lunge exercise is modified into walking lunges. Instead of returning to a standing position after making a static bodyweight lunge on one knee, you reach forward by lunging out on the other leg. The movement is repeated for a predetermined number of repetitions. These lunges are more dynamic than static lunges. They work the leg muscles, the abdominal muscles, the hips, and the glutes. They will help you improve your balance and range of motion.

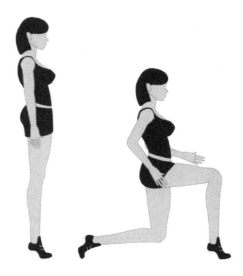

Particulars

Difficulty Level: Advanced.

Equipment Needed: None

Repetitions: 15 repetitions on each leg, total 30 times.

Performing the Exercise

Step 1 (Starting Position): Stand tall with your feet at the shoulder's distance. Keep your hands by the sides of your body or on your hips.

Step 2: Step forward with your left leg, ensure that your weight is pushed into your heel and not the tip of your foot.

Step 3: Bend your left knee and lower it so that it is parallel to the floor. This is the lunge position. Pause for five seconds.

Step 4: Do not move the left leg. Move your right foot forward, and repeat the whole motion. Pause when your right leg is parallel to the floor. This makes one total repetition.

Step 5: Repeat 15 times on each leg till you have performed the exercise 30 times.

Things to Remember

- Keep your body balanced and straight. Do not lean forward or bend too much.
- Make sure your abdominal muscles are engaged during the exercise.
- Don't push your leg too far forward when you lunge because this can make your back curve.
- Push forward till your body feels comfortable, and you can keep your hips and torso straight.

Plank Alternating Knee Tuck Exercise

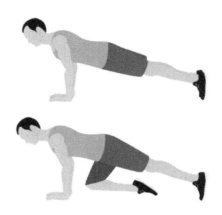

If you're ready to move on to more advanced core training, a plank knee tuck is an excellent option. It requires cross-body movement because it requires all abdominal muscles to complete the exercise and bring the knee to the elbow. Twisting far enough to get the knee entirely over to the opposite arm requires both internal and external oblique muscles. Your oblique muscles become engaged and active. The deep abdominals are engaged, and they aid in bringing the pelvis to a posterior tilt, allowing the knee to meet the opposite limb. As a result, this movement engages all of the abdominal muscles.

This movement also puts less strain on the spine and discs because you're generating more length around the spine than a twisted sit-up where you're on your back.

Particulars

Difficulty Level: Advanced.
Equipment Needed: None.
Repetitions: 5 on each side.

Performing the Exercise

Step 1 (Starting Position): Begin in a full Plank pose, with your palms on the floor and your hands in line with your shoulders.

Step 2: Align yourself to be in a straight line from your shoulders to your feet.

Step 3: Engage your core muscles. You should feel a little tense in them, which means that they are working.

Step 4: Bring your right knee forward across your body to come toward your left elbow.

Step 5: Hold at the top position for a second, and reverse back to your starting position. Keep your body engaged at all times, and do not do any jerking movements.

Step 6: Repeat five times on each side.

Things to Remember

- Take a look at your back and the curve of your spine. Your back should be low enough for you to be able to round it when you lift your lower abdomen. This will allow you to pull your pelvis and your knee to reach your elbow.
- Do not arch your back. This will increase negative pressure on your hip flexors.
- Gently pull your shoulders away from the ears, and keep your eyes positioned over your fingers. Stay forward over the tips of your fingers because this will make your positioning easier.

- Ensure you're working your core muscles (imagine pulling your belly button up to the ceiling) and concentrating on keeping the weight uniformly distributed across your body.

Wall Sit Exercise

Wall sits, also known as wall squats, are an excellent way to increase strength and flexibility in your glutes, calves, quads (front of the thigh), and even your abdominal muscles if you know how to incorporate them. They also engage your concentration and help you to focus on aligning your body for an extended period. This is again an exercise that engages both your mind and body.

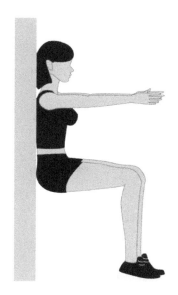

Particulars

Difficulty Level: Advanced.

Equipment Needed: None, but you need to be against a wall.

Repetition/ Time Needed: Hold the position for 15 seconds at the start. Increase slowly, building up to 60 seconds as your endurance grows.

Performing the exercise

Step 1 (Starting Position): Stand with your back flat against a wall. Keep your feet firmly on the ground, at shoulder's distance from each other, and spread it out slowly so that it is two feet in front of the wall.

Step 2: Use your back and bend your knees to slide down the wall. Stop bending your knees at a 90-degree angle. Make sure your abdomen is engaged. Your knees should be directly above your ankles at this stage.

Step 3: Hold this position for 15 seconds, and contract your abdominal muscles.

Step 4: Gently ease back into the starting position, take five breaths, and repeat once more. You can repeat this exercise five times, but stop if you feel exhausted.

Things to Remember

- Make sure your knees are not bouncing, and don't bend down too fast. Control your movements.
- Don't look down. Keep your eyes straight ahead of you.
- If you have trouble keeping your hands to your sides, place them on your thighs, but don't add any pressure.
- Remember to ease into your starting position. Don't jump back into it.

Sit-ups Exercise

Sit-ups are a core exercise that requires you to lie on your back and raise your torso. They reinforce and tone the core-stabilizing abdominal muscles by using your body weight. They strengthen the *rectus abdominis, transverse abdominis*, and obliques, as well as the hip flexors, chest, and neck. They help maintain proper posture by engaging the lower back and gluteal muscles. They also reach more muscles than crunches and static core exercises due to their greater range of motion.

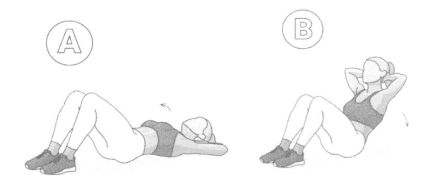

Particulars

Difficulty Level: Advanced.

Equipment Needed: Exercise Mat

Repetitions: Repeat the movement 15 times initially, going up to 30 times as your endurance builds.

Performing the Exercise

Step 1 (Starting Position): Lie flat on your back on the mat, keeping your knees bent and your feet planted on the ground.

Step 2: Draw your chin to your chest so that the back of your neck becomes elongated.

Step 3: Place your fingers at the back of your skull. You can also keep your palms down, flat on the ground.

Step 4: Exhale and lift your upper body to your thighs.

Step 5: Inhale and gently lower your upper body down to the floor.

Things to Remember

- This is a relatively simple exercise, but it will make your abs burn. Just make sure you are not in pain.
- Do not jump up and down. Ease into each motion.
- Adjust your repetitions depending on your level of comfort.

Mountain Climbers Exercise

Mountain climbers are excellent for increasing cardiovascular endurance, aerobic capacity, and stamina. With mountain climbers, you work on several different muscle groups. Your shoulders, arms, and chest work to stabilize your upper body while your abdomen stabilizes the rest of your body. Your quads, which do the primary movements, get a great workout as well. You'll also get heart health benefits and lose calories because it's a cardio workout.

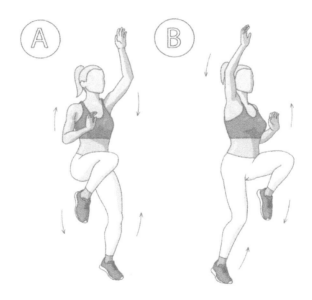

Particulars

Difficulty Level: Advanced.

Equipment Needed: None

Repetitions/ Time Needed: Begin by doing this exercise for 30 seconds. Increase to 60 as your endurance grows.

Performing the Exercise

Step 1 (Starting Position): Stand straight, keeping your arms by your sides and your feet shoulder-width apart.

Step 2: Check your form so that your hands are neutral, your back is smooth.

- Your abs are engaged.
- Your head is straight.

Step 3: Lift your right knee as far as you can towards your chest. Lift your left hand over your head as you lift your right knee in.

Step 4: Switch legs, lifting one knee and pushing the other down.

Step 5: Maintain a neutral hip position and move your knees in and out as far and as quickly as you can with each leg transition, alternate inhaling, and exhaling.

Things to Remember

- Do not bounce on your legs. You will injure yourself if you do this.
- Allow your feet to touch the floor. You won't get the full benefit of the exercise if you fly back and forth.
- Keep your weight balanced and your shoulders in line with your wrists.
- Only do as much as you can take. We aim to strengthen you without hurting your body.

Introduction to Yoga

Yoga has been one of the most beneficial types of exercise for senior citizens. Seniors can strengthen their flexibility and balance, increase their stamina, and improve their mood over time and with suitable classes.

Retirement is a great time to try new things and adopt healthy habits that you might have neglected during your working years. Check out a class if you've never done yoga before, and enjoy some of the benefits of yoga for seniors, such as:

- Bones becoming strengthened: Yoga for seniors may help avoid osteoporosis, a disease that causes fragile or weak bones. As the formation of new bone cannot keep up with the loss of bone mass and density that happens with age, osteoporosis develops.
- Stress reduction: Yoga is a gentle way to release tension in your body, especially in your shoulders and upper back. It alleviates some of the stresses that cause hypertension, resulting in a reduction in the number of drugs used daily. Yoga will also help you relax by lowering your heart rate, blood pressure and making it easier to breathe.

- Better Sleep: Since yoga for seniors can be calming, and many people report sleeping longer and more soundly.
- Balance, stability, agility, and strength improvement: Yoga poses include slow, deliberate movements that can improve balance and movement and help avoid falls. Since falls are some of the leading causes of injury among seniors, yoga will help you gain the mobility to get around more safely.
- Reduce the likelihood of depression: Yoga is a mood enhancer; the combination of movement breathing helps you feel more at ease.
- Effortlessly relieve aches and pains: Yoga can help with aches and pains associated with age, even though you have some physical limitations. Yoga is excellent for people with osteoarthritis because it teaches you how to breathe and relax when coping with chronic pain.

If you're thinking of taking a yoga class, make sure you do your homework first. Many senior centers offer yoga classes designed specifically for seniors. However, below are some simple yet effective yoga techniques you can carry out at home, regardless of your current fitness level.

Chair Yoga

Chair yoga, which was first introduced to the fitness community as a modified form of Hatha Yoga for people with health issues and the elderly, has developed many new fans. With the amount of time people spend sitting at their offices or flying on long flights, there is a push to incorporate more activity and circulation into our everyday routines. Chair yoga can help our bodies by increasing flexibility, relieving cramps and stiffness, and promoting a positive mental attitude.

Chair yoga is a style of yoga that can be performed sitting or standing with the help of a chair. It is ideal for people who can't stand, don't have the agility to switch easily from standing to seated positions and vice versa, or just want a fast break from office work. Chair Yoga is also appropriate for someone immobile, has a physical disability, or has a mental disorder such as dementia or Alzheimer's. Research shows that chair yoga reduces pain, pain interference, and fatigue while also improving gait speed (Park et al., 2017).

Particulars

Difficulty Level: Easy
Equipment Needed: A chair.
Repetitions: Do ten of each variant.

Performing the Exercises

Variant One: Chair Pose

Step 1 (Starting Position): Sit down on a chair, facing a wall if it helps you stay straight. Your back should be aligned, your hands and legs relaxed. Look straight ahead.

Step 2: Bring your hands on your knees, palms facing upward. Connect your thumb to your index finger.

Step 3: Close your eyes, inhale in, and exhale out. Be completely present at the moment.

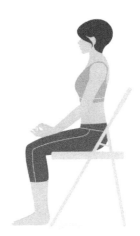

Chair pose

Step 4: Continue breathing in and out ten times.

Variant Two: Sun Salutations

Step 1 (Starting Position): Be seated on a chair, palms on your knees, straight posture, eyes facing forward.

Step 2: Gently raise both your hands above your head in a circular motion, and touch your palms as if you are doing a pranam. Breathe in when you are raising your hands. Breathe out when your palms touch.

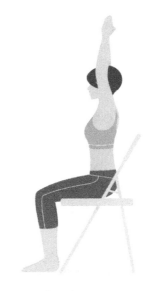

Sun salutations arms

126

Step 3: Gently lower your hands in an anticlockwise motion, and return them to your knees.

Step 4: Repeat ten times.

Variant Three: Forward Bend with Arm Extension

Step 1 (Starting Position): Sit straight on a chair, with your eyes facing forward and back aligned. Keep your hands neutral.

Step 2: Raise your hands in front of you in a vertical motion, and extend them fully. Touch your palms together.

Step 3: Lower your head from your shoulders until your upper torso is in-between your arms. Pause. Breathe in while you lower your head; breathe out once your torso is lowered.

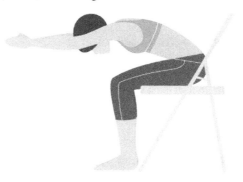

Forward Bend with Arm Extended Forward

Step 4: Gently return to the starting position. Neutralize your arms.

Step 5: Repeat this process ten times.

Variant Four: Forward Bend with Clasped Elbows

Step 1 (Starting Position): Sit straight with your arms by your sides, eyes looking ahead.

Step 2: Raise your hands vertically in front of you, and clasp the left elbow with your right palm and the right elbow with your left palm.

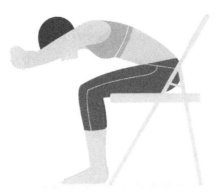

Step 3: Lower your head from your shoulders. Stop when your upper torso is vertically positioned between your arms. Breathe in as you lower yourself, and slowly

Forward Bend with Clasped Elbows

breathe out once you reach the position.

Step 4: Return to the starting position.

Step 5: Repeat ten times.

Things to Remember

- Always keep your back straight. Facing a wall may help you be in a neutral position.
- Remember to keep your eyes in front of you. If you lower them, you might slouch, and if you keep them too high, you may arch your back. This will undo the benefits of the exercise. For maximum benefit, always keep your eyes level.
- Breathing is a critical component of yoga, so always inhale and exhale at every point.

- Challenge yourself. If ten repetitions seem easy, increase them to 15-20. If it seems too much, do five repetitions and increase as you get stronger.

Yoga for Hip and Lower Back Pain

Yoga is a mind-body treatment that's often used for treating back pain and the tension that comes with it. The right poses will help you relax while still strengthening your body. Only a few minutes of yoga practice every day will help you become aware of your body. This will help you notice where you're tense and where your balance is failing you. You can use this knowledge to re-establish harmony and alignment in your life. If you have complaints about lower back pain, it's possible that your hips are to blame. These ten poses will help you strengthen all of the correct muscles and address the root of your pain.

Weak hip muscles often cause lower back pain. Sitting for long periods weakens our abdominals, back muscles, outer hips, and glutes while shortening and tightening our hip flexors, hamstrings, and calves. This muscle imbalance over time is an anterior pelvic tilt, which causes lower back and hip pain.

Start by making it a routine to get up and walk around for a few minutes to combat this issue. Then, as part of your everyday routine, integrate this yoga program. It will help you strengthen your hips, which will help you fight lower back pain. Let's talk about some simple yoga postures you can incorporate into your routine.

Seated Figure Four Exercise

Seated Figure Four is a simple Yoga posture that will help you ease the muscles of your back and hips. It also stretches the piriformis and glutes and relieves stress in the sacral muscles. The piriformis, which stretches from the base of the spine to

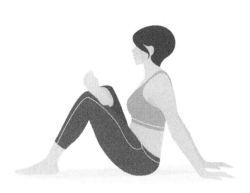

Seated Figure

the top of the femur and aids in hip rotation and stabilization, is the muscle situated deep in your glutes. The piriformis should be kept mobile to avoid inflammation or compression of the sciatic nerve.

Particulars

Difficulty Level: Easy
Equipment Needed: None
Repetitions: 20 repetitions for 2 sets.

Performing the Exercise

Step 1 (Starting Position): Sit on the floor with your knees bent and your feet flat on the floor.
Step 2: Cross your left ankle directly above your knee on top of your right thigh. Make a left-foot flex.

Step 3: Sit tall and inhale. Bring your hips closer to your right foot for a longer stretch.

Step 4: Hold your breath for ten seconds, release, and repeat.

Things to Remember

- Keep your breathing even, and remember to inhale and exhale at every point.
- Make sure you are not feeling uncomfortable with any of the steps. This will undo the purpose of the exercise.
- If you can hold the stretch longer than ten seconds, go for it. But if ten seconds is too much, begin with five.

Frog Yoga Pose Exercise

Frog pose is a yoga pose that can loosen your hip and joint muscles, improve circulation, and improve your posture. After a warm-up that involves a few rounds of sun salutations and lunges or lunge variations to begin opening your hips and preparing for the deeper stretch of frog pose, the frog pose is a perfect step to add to your daily yoga routine. It's particularly beneficial if you're looking for hip-opening benefits while also getting the ability to practice intense, steady, mindful breathing because it's a pose that takes some time to get used to. Frog pose can help to loosen up the hip muscles, which can become tense from repeated motion.

When practiced regularly, the frog pose can help relieve chronic muscle tightness caused by sitting at a desk or driving for long periods.

This pose can help with hip stability and flexibility so that you can sit cross-legged on the floor more comfortably with daily practice.

Particulars

Difficulty Level: Advanced

Equipment Needed: Yoga Mat for comfort

Repetitions: 10 repetitions on each leg.

Performing the Exercise

a) Step 1 (Starting Position):

b) Firstly, start on your hands and knees in a tabletop position.

c) Check that your hands are under your shoulders and that your knees are below your hips.

d) Stay in this position for three to five breaths.

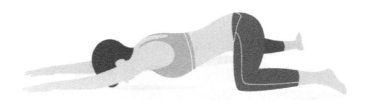

Frog

Step 2: Inhale and, when you exhale, gently lift your right and left knees out to the side, pausing to keep and continue breathing whenever you notice the stretch.

Step 3: Continue to open your hips by turning your feet out to the side and flexing your ankles until your inner feet, ankles, and knees are all touching the floor.

Step 4: Drop yourself to your forearms, keeping your palms flat on the floor or pressed together. If this is too much for you, stay on your palms or place your forearms on the blocks.

Step 5: Stay here and breathe slowly for five to ten breaths, or as long as your body feels comfortable.

Step 6: Return to the tabletop position, slowly sliding your knees closer together to release the frog pose.

Things to Remember

- As with all yoga poses, the breath is an excellent guide. Your breathing will become shorter and more hurried if you drive yourself too far in the stretch. It's a sign that the stretch is right for your body if you can take long, steady, deep breaths.
- Don't let your lower back dip.
- If you're new to this pose or have limitations in your hips or knees, then take this slow.

Crescent Lunge with Prayer Hands

This is a great yoga pose to enhance your overall flexibility. It increases balance and strength, stretches your lungs, back, abdomen, neck, shoulders, and groin. It also strengthens your calves, ankles, and thighs.

Particulars

Difficulty Level: Advanced

Equipment Needed: None

Repetitions: 10 repetitions.

Performing the Exercise

Step 1 (Starting Position): Exhale and take a step forward with your right foot between your hands. Align your right knee over your heel. Then, while keeping your right knee fixed in place, lower your left knee to the floor and slide your left back until you feel a relaxed stretch in your left front thigh.

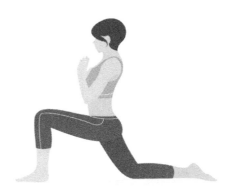

Crescent Lunge on the Knee with Prayer Hands

Step 2: Inhale and straighten your torso. Raise your pubic bone toward your navel and draw your tailbone back toward the floor.

Step 3: Place your hands in front of your chest in a prayer position. Maintain a forward gaze.

Step 4: Take a deep inhalation, and press back to the starting point.

Step 5: Repeat.

Things to Remember

- This yoga pose is advanced and requires a fair amount of balance, so go easy on yourself if it takes time.
- Keep your breathing even.
- Don't arch your back or push too hard. Only do as much as is comfortable.

Yoga for Stiff and Tight Legs

Once you start yoga, you'll realize that many of the poses are difficult not because of the pose itself but because it requires you to hold an immense amount of balance in your legs. The effort can even make your legs shake. This allows your leg muscles to become activated and stronger. In 2014, a study looked at the effects of Hatha Yoga (a variant of yoga for your legs and whole-body) compared with calisthenics in older adults. The study lasted for a year, after which the researchers noted that Hatha Yoga was far more effective in increasing balance and flexibility. With this, let's look at some yoga poses that will make your legs stronger and allow you to move around freely and without fear of falling (Farinatti et al., 2014).

Downward Facing Dog

This is one of the most practiced and basic yoga poses, particularly if you are just starting. It stretches your hamstrings, calves, lower back, and glutes. Its versatility is immense as it works on your shoulders and upper back!

Particulars

Difficulty Level: Easy

Equipment Needed: None

Repetitions: 60-second repetitions done five times.

Performing the Exercise

Step 1 (Starting Position): Start by getting down on your hands and knees. A yoga mat may be used for help.

Step 2: Ensure that your hands are directly under your shoulders and that your feet are directly beneath your hips. Keep your core engaged.

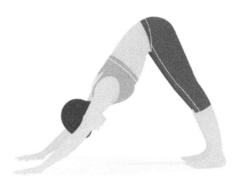

Downward-Facing Dog

Step 3: Take a deep breath and raise yourself off your knees by pressing your weight into your palms, tucking your toes under. Hands should be shoulder-width apart, and heels should be hip-width apart.

Step 4: Lengthen your spine and tailbone. Keep your hands on the ground. On both sides of the body, your weight should be equally distributed.

Step 5: It's perfectly fine if there's any distance between your heels and the floor. Keep this pose for 1 minute, pressing both heels as hard as you can without straining.

Things to Remember

- Examine the toes. From your elbows to your hips, your body should be in a straight line.
- Maintain a straight line with your arms, and do not lock your elbows. Your legs should also be straight.
- Keep your breathing even.

Lunge Pose

This is essentially a low lunge which is beneficial for stretching your quads, hamstrings, and groin. It is a great way to release the tension in your hips.

Particulars

Difficulty Level: Intermediate
Equipment Needed: None
Repetitions: 5 deep breaths on each leg. Repeat on each leg four times.

Performing the Exercise

Step 1 (Starting Position): Go down on all fours in a high plank.

Step 2: Gently and slowly take your left leg ahead and rest it between your hands. Make sure that the right leg is straight backward.

Step 3: Press through your right foot as you press your palms into the floor.

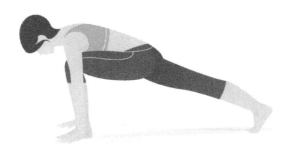

Lunge

Step 4: Take your shoulders back and breathe through your chest, arching forward just a little.

Step 5: Take five deep breaths, and step back with your left leg. Repeat on the other side.

Things to Remember

- This one can be tricky in terms of balance, so don't feel bad if you fumble. Just go slow.
- Keep your breathing even.
- Make sure that your core is engaged and that your legs are working throughout the exercise.

Half-Splits

Half Splits Pose is a gentle way to open up the legs for people of all ages. The calves, hamstrings, and groin are stretched in Half Splits Pose. They also aid in the correction of posture and breathing and the relief of joint pain.

Particulars

Difficulty Level: Intermediate
Equipment Needed: None
Repetitions: Inhale and exhale for 10

Half Splits

seconds on each leg. Repeat on each leg five times.

Performing the Exercise

Step 1 (Starting Position): Start in Downward-Facing Dog, with your palms firmly planted on the floor and your hips lifted high and back. Take a few deep breaths while bending your knees and raising your heels to loosen up the back of your thighs.

Step 2: Move your right foot forward between your hands on an exhale. Lower your left knee to the ground and release the top of your left foot.

Step 3: Straighten your right leg as much as you can by flexing your right foot, coming up onto the heel, and extending your toes back toward you.

Step 4: Maintain a squared-off posture with your hips stacked over your left leg. Inhale to lengthen your back, then exhale and fold your right leg.

Step 5: Draw your right heel back and forward when reaching your chest forward and your shoulder blades down and away from your face.

Step 6: Stay in the pose for ten seconds. Tuck the left toes under, plant the hands and return to Downward-Facing Dog to come out of the pose. When you're ready, switch sides and repeat.

Things to Remember

- If having your hands on the ground feels too difficult, try walking your hands closer to your body or elevating your hands on blocks to reduce the stretch's strength.
- If your back knee is bothering you, consider using a mat and tucking a blanket or towel under it for extra support.

Halfway Lift

Stretch your hamstrings, your upper back, and lengthen your entire spine with this soothing pose. It will require practice and balance, so work your way into it slowly.

Particulars

Difficulty Level: Advanced
Equipment Needed: None
Repetitions: 10-second-deep breaths at the end pose. Repeat exercise ten times.

Performing the Exercise

Step 1 (Starting Position): When you stand, bend over while holding your spine erect. Your feet should be shoulder-width apart or hip-width apart.

Step 2: Place your fingertips next to your feet on the ground. Put your palms to your shins with your fingers pointing straight down.

Step 3: Straighten your arms and raise your shoulders away from your thighs as you inhale. Lengthen your spine and slightly contract your upper back muscles.

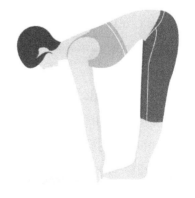

Halfway Lift

141

Step 4: Look ahead slightly without craning your neck.

Step 5: Maintain a solid center and stop rounding the spine. If bending your knees lets you find more length, do so.

Step 6: Release back into the standing forward bend as you exhale.

Things to Remember

- This is difficult only in terms of how much balance it needs. It requires you to bend, so be gentle with yourself.
- If you have trouble bending, do not attempt this pose.

Yoga for Lower Back Tension

Yoga is one of the most common ways to alleviate low back pain and tension. The practice helps strengthen muscles that support the back and neck, including the spinal muscles, which help you bend your spine, the multifidus muscles, which stabilize your vertebrae, and the transverse abdominis, which helps stabilize your spine. Many of the postures in yoga are designed to strengthen the back and abdominal muscles gently. The muscular network of the spine includes back and abdominal muscles, which help the body maintain proper upright posture and movement. Back pain and tension can be significantly minimized or eliminated when these muscles are well-conditioned.

Cow Pose

This simple, straightforward exercise is gentle on your body. It stretches and mobilizes your spine and also stretches shoulders, torso, and neck. It works on the *erector spinae*, triceps, *gluteus maximus*, *rectus abdominis*, and *serratus anterior* muscles.

Particulars

Difficulty Level: Easy

Equipment Needed: None

Repetitions: Breath for 40 seconds at each repetition. Repeat ten times.

Performing the Exercise

Step 1 (Starting Position)

- Begin in a "tabletop" position on your hands and knees.
- Ensure that your knees are directly behind your hips and that your wrists, elbows, and shoulders are in line with the floor.

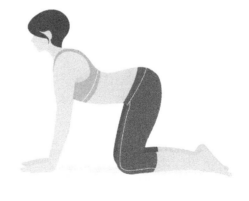

Cow

- With your eyes on the floor, position your head neutrally.

Step 2: Inhale. Raise your chest toward the ceiling as you inhale, allowing your belly to sag to the floor. Lift your brows and look straight ahead.

Step 3: Exhale and return to your hands and knees in a neutral "tabletop" spot.

Step 4: Repeat.

Things to Remember

- Never bounce on this movement because you may end up injuring your neck.
- Be in control of the movement, and keep your eyes focused ahead of you.

The Cat Pose

A variant of the Cow pose, this posture massages the spine and abdominal organs gently. It is a great way to ease your back, particularly if you have chronic back issues.

Particulars

Difficulty Level: Easy
Equipment Needed: None
Repetitions: Breath for 40
seconds at each repetition. Repeat ten times.

Cat

Performing the Exercise

Step 1 (Starting Position):

a) Begin in a "tabletop" position on your hands and knees.
b) Ensure that your knees are directly behind your hips and that your wrists, elbows, and shoulders are in line with the floor.
c) Keep your head in a neutral position with your eyes on the ground.

Step 2: Round your spine toward the ceiling as you exhale, keeping your shoulders and knees in place. Allow your head to fall to the floor, but keep your chin from collapsing into your stomach. Breathe.

Step 3: Return to a neutral "tabletop" position on your hands and knees by inhaling.

Step 4: Repeat.

Things to Remember

- As with the cow pose, keep your eyes fixed, and go through the movement as gently as possible.
- Don't forget to breathe.

Side Body Stretch

The Side Stretch Pose increases energy levels in the body. It relaxes the lower back, mid-back, biceps and triceps, core (abs), hip flexors, Hips, neck, pelvis, Erector spinae, and quadriceps.

Particulars

Difficulty Level: Intermediate

Equipment Needed: None

Repetitions: Hold each rep for 40 seconds. Repeat 20 times.

Performing the Exercise

Step 1 (Starting Position): Sit with your legs crossed. Keep your left hand on the floor, keeping the elbow bent.

Step 2: Extend your right arm upwards and over your head.

Step 3: Move your arms from the right

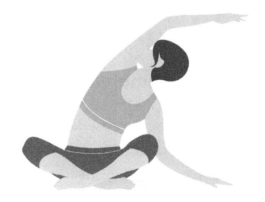

Side body Stretch

to the left until you feel a stretch to your right.

Step 4: Hold here for 40 seconds, return to starting position, and repeat.

Things to Remember

- Don't overextend your right hand. Do it until you feel a good stretch.
- Don't arch your back; your spine should be straight and neutral. Learn from your hips.
- Keep your breathing even.

Seated Twist Pose

This variation of the seated stretch allows you to get a deeper stretch into your muscles while increasing your balance and endurance.

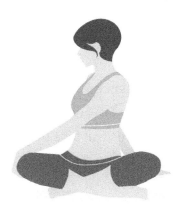

Seated Twist

Particulars

Difficulty Level: Advanced
Equipment Needed: None
Repetitions: Hold each rep for
40 seconds. Repeat 20 times.

Performing the Exercise

Step 1 (Starting Position): Sit with your legs crossed. Keep your left hand on the floor, keeping the elbow bent.

Step 2: Extend your right arm behind and keep extending it until it reaches your left hip. You will find yourself twisting. Twist from your core.

Step 3: Bring your left hand and rest the palm on your right knee.

Step 4: Move yourself from the right to the left until you feel a stretch.

Step 5: Hold here for 40 seconds, return to starting position, and repeat.

Things to Remember

- Don't overextend your arm. Just do as much as is comfortable.
- Remember that the arm you are reaching back has to turn towards the hip of the other side.
- This will take time to master since the exercise is a deep one. Be patient.

Key Points

Before we move on to discussing how you can mix-and-match different exercises into your routine, here are some key points for you!

- Always go at your own pace with the exercises. Don't compare your progress with that of anyone else's.
- Remember that posture is the most important thing when it comes to exercising. You can do a hundred repetitions, but if your posture is poor, it will amount to nothing.
- Keep your breathing even at all times.
- Consult a physician before you begin any exercise plan.
- Ideally, mix exercises from different sections so that you get a full-body workout. We will talk more about this shortly.

CHAPTER 5

Your 7-Day Strength Training Plan

Here is something you need to know- you do not need two-hour long workouts every day to be healthy. This can be counterproductive, exhausting you and making you give up in a few days. Instead, we aim to induce short bursts of high-intensity training, combining exercises discussed in chapter 4. Individual fitness programs should be adjusted based on their usual physical activity, physical function, health status, exercise reactions, and specified goals.

Adults who cannot achieve the exercise goals outlined here will still benefit from exercising in less than prescribed quantities. Even in physically active adults, there are health benefits to minimizing overall time spent in sedentary pursuits and interspersing frequent, brief bursts of standing and physical activity between periods of sedentary activity.

In both healthy people and people with cardiometabolic diseases, as few as three HIIT (high-intensity interval training) sessions a week, involving few minutes of intense exercise, including warm-up, and cool-down, has been shown to improve exercise tolerance, health, and physical strength (Gillen et al., 2014). Research conducted in 2013 aimed to study the effect of high-intensity interval training in older adults. Participants increased their physical health significantly and improved their physical activity and health-related quality of life. The research suggested that exercise therapy should be used to care for older adults at risk of functional deterioration (Brovold et al., 2013).

So, if you find that time is a constraint or that the only thing stopping you from partaking in physical activity is the fear of how strenuous it has to be, you don't have to be worried any longer. With this in mind, let's discuss your 7-day exercise plan. Each day will comprise 7-minute exercise routines. One routine will increase your strength, while the other will focus on meditative techniques drawn from yoga. The latter will help you build a healthy mind-body relationship while also increasing your flexibility.

If you are starting, limit the number of exercises that need to be learned, and for the first few weeks, stick with what you know. This will simplify the training schedules. For instance, if there are seven exercises that you don't know, choose four, learn them well on day one, and repeat them for ten days before attempting to learn something new. The workouts are interchangeable, and you can replace one routine for another to keep things interesting. I suggest beginning with the easy exercises and low-intensity training and building up to more advanced moves. Done correctly, these exercises will help you increase your routine functionality. We will emphasize building your strength and balance so that you are at less risk of falls and bone deterioration. We will also incorporate warm-ups and cool-downs to help your muscles breathe.

Reminder: You will perform each of these sessions two times every day. Each session lasts for 7 minutes. However, my experience shows that only one session lasting for 7 minutes can make a significant difference. If you wish to carry out only one session, then that is perfectly fine. As you progress and your body strengthens, you can add the second session as well. For this, my advice would be to pace the workouts - once in the daytime and once in the evening.

Day 1

Warm-Up

Stand still at a quiet corner of your room where you will perform the workout. Do each stretch for 20 seconds. Try not to pause in-between since we aim to get the muscles warm in a short period.

Calf Stretch: 20 seconds.
Triceps Stretch: 20 seconds.
Neck Stretch: 20 seconds.
Hamstring Stretch: 20 seconds.

Strength Workout 1:

- Perform each exercise for 40 seconds.
- Take a 10-second pause between exercises, but do not sit down.
- Stand or move around and return to the exercise.

Exercise 1: Hip Raise, perform for 40 seconds. Try your best not to pause during the exercise.

Duration: 10-second break.

Exercise 2: Dumbbell Shoulder Shrug, perform for 40 seconds.

Duration: 10-second break.

Exercise 3: Dumbbell Overhead Shoulder Press, perform for 40 seconds.

Duration: 10-second break.

Exercise 4: 90-90 crunch, perform for 40 seconds.

Cool Down:

Perform the cool-down stretches for 30 seconds each. Try not to pause between them.

Side Body Stretch: 30 seconds

Chair Yoga Variant 2 (Sun Salutations): 30 seconds

Meditative Workout 1

This is designed to help you gain balance, relaxation, and flow. We will target your breathing with this exercise. Perform this exercise for 90 seconds. For the first day, we will practice alternate-nostril breathing.

Step 1: Bend your pointer and middle fingers into the palm of your hand, leaving your thumb, ring finger, and pinky extended. Close your eyes.

Step 2: To start, take a few deep breaths in and out.

Step 3: Through your thumb, close your right nostril.

Step 4: Take a deep breath through your left nostril.

Step 5: Using your ring finger, close your left nostril.

Step 6: Exhale from your right nostril when you open it. Repeat for 90 seconds.

The workout is complete.

Day 2

Warm-Up

Calf Stretch: 20 seconds.

Triceps Stretch: 20 seconds.

Quadriceps Stretch: 20 seconds

Overhead Triceps Stretch: 20 seconds.

Strength Workout 2

Perform each exercise for 40 seconds.

Exercise 1: Dumbbell Curl, perform for 40 seconds. Do not pause when you are performing the activity.

10-second break.

Exercise 2: Dumbbell Overhead Shoulder Press, perform for 40 seconds.

10-second break.

Exercise 3: Leg Raise, perform for 40 seconds.

10-second break.

Exercise 4: Triceps Dips, perform for 40 seconds.

Cool Down

Perform the cool-down stretches for 30 seconds each. Do not pause between them.

Frog Pose: 30 seconds

Chair Yoga Variant 1 (Chair Pose): 30 seconds

Meditative Workout 2

This exercise encourages you to breathe from your belly. Perform this for 90 seconds.

Step 1: Sit or lie down. Try to sit in a chair, sitting cross-legged, or lying down on your back with a small cushion between your knees and head.

Step 2: Next step, place one hand on your upper chest and the other on your stomach, just below your ribcage.

Step 3: Allow your stomach to relax without squeezing or clenching your muscles to push it inward.

Step 4: Slowly inhale through your nose. The air should travel through your nose and down, causing your stomach to rise with one hand and fall inward with the other (toward your spine).

Step 5: Slowly exhale with slightly pursed lips. Keep an eye on the hand on your face, which should be fairly still. Repeat this movement for 90 seconds.

The workout is complete.

Day 3

Warm-Up

Find a quiet spot and do each activity for 20 seconds. Do not pause in-between warm-up movements.

Inner-thigh Stretch: 20 seconds.

Shoulder Stretch: 20 seconds.

Neck Stretch: 20 seconds.

Hamstring Stretch: 20 seconds.

Strength Workout 3

Perform each exercise for 40 seconds. Take a 10-second pause between exercises.

Exercise 1: Single leg lift, perform for 40 seconds.

10-second break.

Exercise 2: Hip Raises, perform for 40 seconds.

10-second break.

Exercise 3: Dumbbell Curl, perform for 40 seconds.

10-second break.

Exercise 4: Dumbbell Floor Chest Press, perform for 40 seconds.

Cool Down

Perform the cool-down stretches for 30 seconds each. Do not pause.

Crescent Lunge on Knee with Prayer Hands Stretch: 30 seconds

Chair Yoga Variant 3 (Forward Bend with Arm Extension): 30 seconds

Meditative Workout 3

Box breathing, also known as four-square breathing, is an easy technique to learn and master. This style of paced breathing is already familiar to you if you've ever found yourself inhaling and exhaling to the beat of music.

Step 1: Breathe out and count to 4.

Step 2: Inhale for four counts.

Step 3: Exhale and restart the pattern. Repeat for 90 seconds. The workout is complete.

Day 4

Warm-Up

Find a quiet spot and do each activity for 20 seconds. Do not pause in-between warm-up movements.

Inner-thigh Stretch: 20 seconds.

Calf Stretch: 20 seconds.

Neck Stretch: 20 seconds.

Shoulder Stretch: 20 seconds.

Strength Workout 4

Perform every exercise for 40 seconds. Take a 10-second pause between them.

Exercise 1: Single leg lift, perform for 40 seconds.

10-second break.

Exercise 2: Single-leg Raises, perform for 40 seconds.

10-second break.

Exercise 3: Triceps Dips, perform for 40 seconds.

10-second break.

Exercise 4: Dumbbell Floor Chest Press, perform for 40 seconds.

Cool Down

Perform the cool-down stretches for 30 seconds each. Do not pause.

Frog Pose: 30 seconds

Chair Yoga Variant 1 (Sun Salutations): 30 seconds

Meditative Workout 4

Coherent breathing, also known as resonance breathing, will help you relax and reduce anxiety.

Step 1: Close your eyes and lie down.

Step 2: Breath in slowly through your nose, mouth closed, for six seconds. Don't overfill your lungs, and be in control of your breathing.

Step 3: Enable your breath to leave your body slowly and gently for six seconds, without pushing it.

Step 4: Repeat till 90 seconds is over.

The workout is complete.

Day 5

Warm-Up:

Find a quiet spot and do every exercise for 20 seconds. Do not pause till the warm-up is complete.

Inner-thigh Stretch: 20 seconds.

Calf Stretch: 20 seconds.

Quadriceps Stretch: 20 seconds.

Hamstring Stretch: 20 seconds.

Strength Workout 5

Each exercise should be completed in 40 seconds. Between exercises, take a 10-second pause, but do not stop when you are performing them.

Exercise 1: Bird Dog, perform for 40 seconds.

10-second break.

Exercise 2: Single-leg Deadlift, perform for 40 seconds.

10-second break.

Exercise 3: Two-arm Bent-over Row, perform for 40 seconds.

10-second break.

Exercise 4: Side Plank, perform for 40 seconds.

Cool Down

Perform each cool-down stretches for 30 seconds. Do not stop between them.

Downward Facing Dog: 30 seconds

Chair Yoga Variant 4 (Forward Bend with Clasped Elbows): 30 seconds

Meditative Workout 5

We will perform the 4-7-8 breathing exercise for this routine, which serves as a natural nervous system relaxant. It's best to start by doing the exercise while seated with your back straight. However, once you've gotten used to the breathing exercise, you can do it while lying in bed.

Step 1: For the duration of the exercise, press the tip of your tongue against the ridge of tissue behind your upper front teeth.

Step 2: Make a *whoosh* sound by fully exhaling through your mouth.

Step 3: Close your mouth and inhale softly through your nose, counting till 4.

Step 4: Hold your breath for seven counts.

Step 5: At count 8, exhale fully through your mouth.

The workout is complete.

Day 6

Warm-Up

Perform the warm-up movements without pausing in-between.

Inner-thigh Stretch: 20 seconds.

Shoulder Stretch: 20 seconds.

Neck Stretch: 20 seconds.

Hamstring Stretch: 20 seconds.

Strength Workout 6

Complete each exercise in 40 seconds, with 10 second rest periods in between.

Exercise 1: Air Squats, perform for 40 seconds.

10-second break.

Exercise 2: Fire Hydrants, perform for 40 seconds.

10-second break.

Exercise 3: Crunches, perform for 40 seconds.

10-second break.

Exercise 4: Walking Lunges, perform for 40 seconds.

Cool Down

Perform each cool-down stretches for 30 seconds without any pauses.

Cow Pose: 30 seconds

Seated Twist: 30 seconds

Meditative Workout 6

Another beneficial deep breathing technique is lion's breath. It may aid in the relaxation of facial and jaw muscles and the improvement of cardiovascular functions. The exercise is best done in a relaxed sitting position with your hands on your knees or the floor, leaning forward slightly.

Step 1: Extend your fingers as far as they can go.

Step 2: Inhale slowly and deeply through your nose.

Step 3: Extend your tongue down into your chin by opening your mouth wide and sticking it out.

Step 4: Forcefully exhale, bringing your breath across the root of your tongue.

Step 5: Create a "ha" sound from deep inside your abdomen when exhaling.

Step 6: Breathe normally, and repeat.

The workout is complete.

Day 7

Warm-Up: Perform the warm-up movements without any pauses.

Inner-thigh Stretch: 20 seconds.

Shoulder Stretch: 20 seconds.

Quadriceps Stretch: 20 seconds.

Calf Stretch: 20 seconds.

Strength Workout 7

Complete each exercise in 40 seconds, with 10-second gaps between each.

Exercise 1: Single Leg Bridge, perform for 40 seconds.
10-second break.

Exercise 2: Mountain Climbers, perform for 40 seconds.
10-second break.

Exercise 3: Dumbbell Split Squat, perform for 40 seconds.
10-second break.

Exercise 4: Plank Alternating Knee Tuck, perform for 40 seconds.

Cool Down

Perform the cool-down stretches for 30 seconds with no rest in-between.

Cat Pose: 30 seconds
Side-body Stretch: 30 seconds

Meditative Workout 7

For day seven, we will acquaint ourselves with mindfulness meditation. Focusing on your breathing and taking your attention to the moment without allowing your mind to wander to the past or future is what mindfulness meditation entails.

Step 1: Choose a soothing focus to repeat silently as you inhale or exhale, such as calm words that include *"inhale positivity, exhale tension."*

Step 2: Relax and let go. Take a deep breath and gently bring your mind back to the present moment when you find your mind has wandered. Be engaged in this for 90 seconds.

The workout is complete.

Well done for making it this far! You are someone who is genuinely committed to seeking out positive change and ways to live well. We are almost done, but before we conclude, let's look at some quick reminders.

Key Points

- Stick to the time divisions given. These workouts will take seven minutes of your daily schedules and no more.

- Remember the breathing patterns advised, particularly for meditation exercises.

- Try to catch your breath. Try to never pause during warm-ups or cool downs because that will interfere with the rate at which your body warms or cools- and we need to optimize both to finish the workout in 7 minutes.

- Make sure to consult your physician before you begin.

- Once you become more comfortable, alternate between these exercises and the ones we discussed in chapter 4; keep the time frames mentioned.

Conclusion

As we age, many of us become complacent with our lives. Many people aged 65 spend hours sitting around or doing nothing, making them the most sedentary age group. Compared to the general population, they end up paying a high price for their inactivity, with higher rates of falls, obesity, heart disease, and early death. It's even more important to stay involved as you get older if you want to stay safe and preserve your freedom.

If you don't remain involved, all of the activities you've always enjoyed and taken for granted can become more difficult. You can find it challenging to engage in simple pleasures such as playing with your grandchildren, walking to the store, participating in recreational activities, and socializing with friends. You can begin to experience aches and pains that you have never experienced before, as well as a lack of energy to go out. You may also be more prone to dropping. This will make it difficult for you to look after yourself and do the things you love.

Exercise is an essential component of virtually everyone's daily wellbeing. This is also valid for senior citizens. By now, you will know that you should be involved in physical activity as much as possible.

There are several advantages to exercising as a senior, including boosting your stamina, helping you maintain your balance and equilibrium, boosting energy, preventing or delaying the onset of lifestyle and neurodegenerative disorders, and enhancing cognitive function.

It is safe to exercise for most adults over the age of 65. Patients with chronic illnesses should exercise safely as well. Heart disease, high blood pressure, arthritis, and diabetes are among them. In reality, exercise can help with a lot of these issues. As I mentioned, ask your doctor if you're not sure if exercise is healthy for you or if you're currently inactive. If a particular activity is not suitable for you, you can easily replace it with something else. We have also talked about ways to stretch your muscles and relax your body so that you will feel reinvigorated at the end of each workout. Treat the workouts as medicine for your soul, as ways to live your life on your terms.

Once you have the green light, use this book to the best of your abilities. Take notes, add modifications, and make it your workout journal, if you will. The book has been designed to help you realize your fitness goals to go into old age, feeling like you are in control of your life. There is nothing more valuable than that. Remember that consistency is key. My book does not ask too much of you, but it does need you to show up for 7 minutes every day. 7 minutes of devotion to your body and mind, both of which have carried you this far.

Remember that along with all this, nutrition also has a vital role to play, so don't neglect it. We often lose the will to eat as we grow old and consume whatever comes our way. It is more important for us to maintain our nutrition as we age. It can be a great tool in preventing the early onset of dementia and preserving your bones. Blood pressure and hypertension are common problems that come our way, so modify your diet to reduce your sodium intake. Consume plenty of green vegetables, lentils, and vegetables red and yellow, like red and yellow peppers. Reduce your intake of meat. If you enjoy non-vegetarian food, rely on fish which is good for your heart. Avoid as much as you can on deep-fried food. Wherever possible, consume home-cooked food. You may think that food coming from stores is healthy as long as they come in forms like salads. Still, you don't know what is in them- whether the veggies are fresh, whether the dressing is safe, how much sodium is in it, whether there are any preservatives added to maintain taste and texture, and more such questions. To stay safe, eat food that you are familiar with. And supplement your diet with the exercises we have covered.

Read and look through the exercises as many times as you need. Enlist friends and family to perform them with you, but get started. Don't keep anything for tomorrow because the sooner you start, the better tomorrow becomes. A day spent waiting is a day wasted in poor health. If you have days where you feel tired or unwilling to workout, remember the reasons why you are doing this- for preserving your independence, for not having to rely on anyone to survive, for not depending on people as if they are crutches. If there is a way to be around people without this dependency, isn't it a fantastic way to live? And if you still feel tired, go out and take a walk. Spend some time reorienting yourself, and come back with a fresh mind. Remember that slips happen, and they are natural. So don't blame yourself if you have one bad day. Just pick up on the next day and begin from where you left off. Your journey is the sum of all the work you put in, and one bad day is not the beginning or the end of it.

I am so happy that you have reached the end of my book. I truly hope that it gives you the push you need to live the life that you deserve. I wish you the very best for your forthcoming journey. I have included several resources such as seven-day exercise logs, key exercise tables, and much more that you can freely download from **www.7minutestraining.com**

.

PLEASE LEAVE ME A REVIEW!

If you liked this book, please write a review on Amazon.
Your reviews will help me to know that my work has benefited
you, helping me develop further books.

Customer reviews

★★★★★ 5 out of 5

4 global ratings

5 star		100%
4 star		0%
3 star		0%
2 star		0%
1 star		0%

˅ How are ratings calculated?

Review this product

Share your thoughts with other customers

Write a customer review

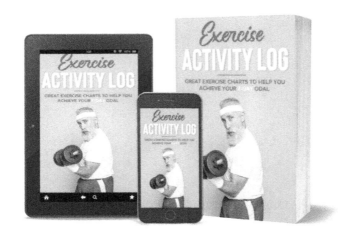

A SPECIAL GIFT TO OUR READERS!

Included with your purchase of this book is our **Exercise Activity Log** that will help you achieve your 7-day strength training goal. This is a great way to keep a record of your training.

USE THE LINK:
www.7minutestraining.com

OR SCAN THE QR CODE

JOIN OUR ONLINE SUPPORT GROUP

To maximize the value of your strength training, I highly encourage you to join our tight-knit community on Facebook, where you will be able to ask questions and get tips on your training.

USE THE LINK:

https://www.facebook.com/groups/strengthtrainingforseniors

OR SCAN THE QR CODE

REFERENCES

Booth, F. W., Roberts, C. K., & Laye, M. J. (2012). Lack of exercise is a major cause of chronic diseases. *Comprehensive Physiology*, *2*(2), 1143–1211. https://doi.org/10.1002/cphy.c110025

Brovold, T., Skelton, D. A., & Bergland, A. (2013). Older adults recently discharged from the hospital: effect of aerobic interval exercise on health-related quality of life, physical fitness, and physical activity. *Journal of the American Geriatrics Society*, *61*(9), 1580–1585. https://doi.org/10.1111/jgs.12400

Butler-Browne, G., Mouly, V., Bigot, A., & Trollet, C. (2018). *How Muscles Age, and How Exercise Can Slow It*. The Scientist.

Darr KC, Schultz E. Exercise-induced satellite cell activation in growing and mature skeletal muscle. *J Appl Physiol* 1987;**63**:1816–1821.

Douka, S., Zilidou, V. I., Lilou, O., & Manou, V. (2019). Traditional Dance Improves the Physical Fitness and Well-Being of the Elderly. *Frontiers in Aging Neuroscience*.

Effects of obesity and exercise: Is obesity a mental health issue? The Harvard Mental Health Letter investigates. (2014). Harvard

Health Publishing.
https://www.health.harvard.edu/press_releases/obesity_exerc
ise_and_effects

Exercise after Age 70. (2019). Harvard Women's Health Watch.
https://www.health.harvard.edu/staying-
healthy/exercise_after_age_70

Fabian, D. & Flatt, T. (2011) The Evolution of Aging. *Nature
Education Knowledge* 3(10):9

Farinatti, P. T., Rubini, E. C., Silva, E. B., & Vanfraechem, J. H.
(2014). Flexibility of the elderly after one-year practice of
yoga and calisthenics. *International journal of yoga therapy,
24*, 71–77.

Garber, C. E., Blissmer, B., Deschenes, M. R., Franklin, B. A.,
Lamonte, M. J., Lee, I. M., Nieman, D. C., Swain, D. P., &
American College of Sports Medicine (2011). American
College of Sports Medicine position stand. Quantity and
quality of exercise for developing and maintaining
cardiorespiratory, musculoskeletal, and neuromotor fitness
in apparently healthy adults: guidance for prescribing
exercise. *Medicine and science in sports and exercise, 43*(7),
1334–1359. https://doi.org/10.1249/MSS.0b013e318213fefb

Gillen, J. B., & Gibala, M. J. (2014). Is high-intensity interval training
a time-efficient exercise strategy to improve health and
fitness?. *Applied physiology, nutrition, and metabolism =
Physiologie appliquee, nutrition et metabolisme, 39*(3), 409–
412. https://doi.org/10.1139/apnm-2013-0187

Griffin, R. M. (2021). *Myths About Exercise and Older Adults.* Compass by WebMD. https://www.webmd.com/healthy-aging/features/exercise-older-adults#1

Hamilton, A. (2021). *Older athletes: don't get sore, get faster!* Sports Performance Bulletin. https://www.sportsperformancebulletin.com/endurance-training/masters/older-athletes-dont-get-sore-get-faster/

Klentrou, P., Slack, J., Roy, B., & Ladouceur, M. (2007). Effects of exercise training with weighted vests on bone turnover and isokinetic strength in postmenopausal women. *Journal of aging and physical activity, 15*(3), 287–299. https://doi.org/10.1123/japa.15.3.287

King, A.C. (2001). Interventions to promote physical activity in older adults. *The Journal of Gerontology: Series A,* 56A, 36-46.

Kyuwoong Kim, Seulggie Choi, Seo Eun Hwang, Joung Sik Son, Jong-Koo Lee, Juhwan Oh, Sang Min Park. Changes in exercise frequency and cardiovascular outcomes in older adults. *European Heart Journal,* 2019; DOI: 10.1093/eurheartj/ehz768

Lee C. Attitudes, knowledge, and stages of change: a survey of exercise patterns in older Australian women. *Health Psychology.* 1993;12: 476–480

Lees, F.D., Clark, P.G., Nigg, C.R., & Newman, P. (2005). Barriers to exercise behavior among older adults: a focus-group study. *Journal of Aging & Physical Activity,* 13, 23-13.

http://journals.humankinetics.com/AcuCustom/Sitename/D
ocuments/DocumentItem/4512.pdf.

Martins, R., Coelho E Silva, M., Pindus, D., Cumming, S., Teixeira,
A., & Veríssimo, M. (2011). Effects of strength and aerobic-
based training on functional fitness, mood and the
relationship between fatness and mood in older adults. *The
Journal of sports medicine and physical fitness*, *51*(3), 489–
496.

Mathews, A.E., Laditka, S.B., Laditka, J.N., Wilcox, S., Corwin, S.J.,
Liu, R., Friedman, D.B., Hunter, R., Tseng, W., & Logsdon,
R.G. (2010). Older adults' perceived physical activity enablers
and barriers: a multicultural perspective. *Journal of Aging &
Physical Activity,* 18, 119-140.

Melov, S., Tarnopolsky, M. A., Beckman, K., Felkey, K., & Hubbard,
A. (2007). Resistance exercise reverses aging in human
skeletal muscle. *PloS one*, *2*(5), e465.
https://doi.org/10.1371/journal.pone.0000465

N.A. Duggal et al. (2018), "Major features of immune senescence,
including reduced thymic output, are ameliorated by high
levels of physical activity in adulthood," *Aging Cell*, 17:e12750

Nicholas T. Broskey, Chiara Greggio, Andreas Boss, Marie Boutant,
Andrew Dwyer, Leopold Schlueter, Didier Hans, Gerald
Gremion, Roland Kreis, Chris Boesch, Carles Canto,
Francesca Amati, Skeletal Muscle Mitochondria in the
Elderly: Effects of Physical Fitness and Exercise Training, *The
Journal of Clinical Endocrinology & Metabolism*, Volume 99,

Issue 5, 1 May 2014, Pages 1852–1861,
https://doi.org/10.1210/jc.2013-3983

Park, J., McCaffrey, R., Newman, D., Liehr, P., & Ouslander, J. G. (2017). A Pilot Randomized Controlled Trial of the Effects of Chair Yoga on Pain and Physical Function Among Community-Dwelling Older Adults With Lower Extremity Osteoarthritis. *Journal of the American Geriatrics Society*, 65(3), 592–597. https://doi.org/10.1111/jgs.14717

Puetz, T. W., Flowers, S. S., & O'Connor, P. J. (2008). A randomized controlled trial of the effect of aerobic exercise training on feelings of energy and fatigue in sedentary young adults with persistent fatigue. *Psychotherapy and psychosomatics*, *77*(3), 167–174. https://doi.org/10.1159/000116610

Robinson, L., Smith, M., & Segal, J. (2020). *Senior Exercise and Fitness Tips*. HelpGuide.Org. https://www.helpguide.org/articles/healthy-living/exercise-and-fitness-as-you-age.htm#:~:text=People who exercise tend to,mobility%2C flexibility%2C and balance.

Rosenberg, D. E., Bombardier, C. H., Hoffman, J. M., & Belza, B. (2011). Physical activity among persons aging with mobility disabilities: shaping a research agenda. *Journal of aging research*, *2011*, 708510. https://doi.org/10.4061/2011/708510

R. Sreekumar et al., (2002). "Gene expression profile in skeletal muscle of type 2 diabetes and the effect of insulin treatment," *Diabetes*, 51:1913–20.

Sarwer, D. B., & Polonsky, H. M. (2016). The Psychosocial Burden of Obesity. *Endocrinology and metabolism clinics of North America*, 45(3), 677–688. https://doi.org/10.1016/j.ecl.2016.04.016

S. Melov et al (2007). "Resistance exercise reverses aging in human skeletal muscle," *PLOS ONE*, 2:e465.

Stewart, K. J., Turner, K. L., Bacher, A. C., DeRegis, J. R., Sung, J., Tayback, M., & Ouyang, P. (2003). Are fitness, activity, and fatness associated with health-related quality of life and mood in older persons?. *Journal of cardiopulmonary rehabilitation*, 23(2), 115–121. https://doi.org/10.1097/00008483-200303000-00009

Study reveals performing light physical activity prevents major mobility disability among elderly. (2020). Asia News International. https://www.aninews.in/news/lifestyle/culture/study-reveals-performing-light-physical-activity-prevents-major-mobility-disability-among-elderly20200614132012/

Vainionpää, A., Korpelainen, R., Sievänen, H., Vihriälä, E., Leppäluoto, J., & Jämsä, T. (2007). Effect of impact exercise and its intensity on bone geometry at weight-bearing tibia and femur. *Bone*, 40(3), 604–611. https://doi.org/10.1016/j.bone.2006.10.005

Yamada Y, Noriyasu R, Kimura M, et al. Association between lifestyle and physical activity level in the elderly: a study using doubly labeled water and simplified physical activity record.

European Journal Of Applied Physiology [serial online]. October 2013;113(10):2461-2471. Available from: MEDLINE Complete, Ipswich, MA. Accessed April 24, 2017.

Made in United States
North Haven, CT
19 February 2022

16282159R00102